Enfield Libraries

RZ

**Transferred to RZ
May 2003**

Please remember that this item will attract overdue charges if not returned by the latest date stamped above. You may renew it in person, by telephone or by post quoting the bar code number and your library card number.

www.enfield.gov.uk

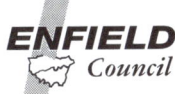

Historic Books on
Veterinary Science and Animal Husbandry
===

SNAPE's
Purging Pill
FOR
HORSES:

With His

Cordial Pouder, and *Ointments*.

Prepared for the Good of the *Publick*, but more especially for the *Gentry* in the remote parts of this Kingdom.

By *Andrew Snape*, Author of *the Anatomy of an Horse*, and Serjeant Farrier to their present Majesties.

LONDON,
Printed in the Year 1692.

SCIENCE MUSEUM

Historic Books on Veterinary Science and Animal Husbandry

The Comben Collection in the Science Museum Library

Pauline Dingley

LONDON: HMSO

© Trustees of the Science Museum 1992

First published 1992

ISBN 0 11 290511 0

British Library Cataloguing in Publication Data

A CIP catalogue record for this book is available from the British Library

HMSO publications are available from:
HMSO Publications Centre
(Mail, fax and telephone orders only)
PO Box 276, London, SW8 5DT
Telephone orders 071-873 9090
General enquiries 071-873 0011
(queuing system in operation for both numbers)
Fax orders 071-873 8200

HMSO Bookshops
49 High Holborn, London, WC1V 6HB
(counter service only)
071-873 0011   Fax 071-873 8200
258 Broad Street, Birmingham, B1 2HE
021-643 3740   Fax 021-643 6510
Southey House, 33 Wine Street, Bristol, BS1 2BQ
0272 264306   Fax 0272 294515
9-21 Princess Street, Manchester, M60 8AS
061-834 7201   Fax 061-833 0634
16 Arthur Street, Belfast, BT1 4GD
0232 238451   Fax 0232 235401
71 Lothian Road, Edinburgh, EH3 9AZ
031-228 4181   Fax 031-229 2734

HMSO's Accredited Agents
(see Yellow Pages)

and through good booksellers

Typeset in Baskerville from Pagemaker 4.0 at the Science Museum
Printed in the UK for HMSO
Dd 291799 C5 56-5419 29254 11/92

Contents

List of illustrations   7

Foreword   9

Acknowledgements   10

Introduction   11

References cited   13

Cataloguing conventions   15

Historic books   19

Reference books   167

List of illustrations

Snape, A. Snape's purging pill for horses. 1692 (575)   Frontispiece
Plagiarism in veterinary anatomy, 1598-1806, from Ruini (541), Snape (573), Gibson (289) and Burke (125)   16 and 17
A.S. The gentleman's compleat jockey. 1696 (1)   20
A.S. The husbandman's instructor. [168-?] (4)   21
Allen, M. The farrier's assistant. 1737 (11)   23
Baret, M. An hipponomie. 1618 (29)   26
Bartlet, J. The gentleman's farriery. 1777 (36)   29
Blaine, D. A concise description of the distemper in dogs. 1806 (66)   34
Bradstreet, J. The farmers request. 1730 (103)   40
Breckon, H. A cow doctor. 1820 (104)   41
Breckon, H. A sheep doctor. 1820 (105)   42
Clark, C. An exposure of abuses and malpractices at ... the Royal Veterinary College. 1829 (157)   50
Clater, F. Every man his own farrier. 1783 (163)   52
Clifford, C. The schoole of horsmanship. 1585 (171)   54
Corte, C. The art of riding. 1584 (196)   58
Crawshey, J. The good husband's jewel. [17--?] (202)   60
Diderot, D. Maréchal ferrant. [1769] (223)   64
E.R. The experienced farrier. 1678 (236)   67
Ellis, W. Every farmer his own farrier. 1759 (244)   69
Estienne, C. Maison rustique. 1616 (246)   70
Fitzherbert, J. The boke of husbandry. 1534 (261)   73
Forester, B. The pocket farrier. [1770?] (268)   75
Freeman, S. The farrier's vade mecum. 1772 (270)   77
The Gentleman or traveller's pocket-farrier. 1732 (282)   79
Gibson, W. The farrier's new guide. 1738 (288)   81
Grisone, F. Ordini di cavalcare. 1584 (304)   84
Halfpenny, J. The gentleman's jocky. 1671 (307)   86
The Horseman and traveller's perfect director. [17--] (340)   91
Jeffray, J. An address to the public. 1786 (356)   94
Lane, J. The principles of English farriery vindicated. 1800 (374)   98
Leeming, J. Every man his own farrier. 1771 (395)   102
Markham, G. Markhams maister-peece. 1610 (434)   108 and 109
Markham, G. The perfect horseman. 1656 (442)   112
Morgan, N. The perfection of horse-manship. 1609 (465)   116
Morgan, N. The horse-mans honour. 1620 (466)   118
Ruini, C. Anatomia del cavallo. 1618 (541)   130
Sainbel, C.V. de. The works of Charles Vial de Sainbel. 1795 (547)   132

Scott's Tables. 1828 (554)   135
The Shepherd's guide. [1819] (561)   137
Sinclair, A.G. Critical observations and remarks. 1792 (567)   139
Stubbs, G. The anatomy of the horse. 1766 (600)   144
Taplin, W. Taplin's Multum in parvo. 1796 (615)   148
Vegetius Renatus. Of the distempers of horses. 1748 (646)   154
Veterinary College, London. A brief examination of the views. 1795 (647)   155
White, J. The anatomy and physiology of the horse's foot. 1801 (662)   158
Wyke, I. The English and Welsh cattle doctor. [1812] (693)   163
Young, A. An essay on the management of hogs. 1769 (702)   165

Foreword

The Comben Collection of historic books on veterinary science and animal husbandry now forms a new and important part of the rare books collection in the Science Museum Library. Its acquisition was made possible in 1987 by grants from the National Heritage Memorial Fund, the Wolfson Foundation at the British Library, the Pilgrim Trust, and the Friends of the National Libraries supplemented by the Museum's own Purchase Fund.

Unique in its scope and richness, the Comben Collection complements the Museum's substantial holding of three-dimensional objects associated with the history of veterinary science, part of which is now displayed in a permanent *Veterinary History Gallery* adjacent to the area in the Science Museum devoted to medical history – the Wellcome Museum for the History of Medicine.

We are most grateful to Norman Comben not only for the dedication and enthusiasm with which he built the collection, but also for the continuing interest and support during the preparation of the catalogue and for the financial assistance that has allowed it to be published in its present form.

Through the influence of Norman Comben – and that of others – there is growing interest in a subject whose long history was recently marked by the bicentenary of the establishment, in 1791, of the first veterinary college in the British Isles – the (now Royal) Veterinary College in London. We hope that a detailed catalogue produced at this time will be of lasting value to veterinary historians and other collectors, as well as to librarians and to the antiquarian book trade.

Neil Cossons
Director
National Museum of Science & Industry
1992

Acknowledgements

I should like to acknowledge the work of Judit Brody, formerly with the Science Museum Library, in preparing the initial entries for the library catalogue. I am grateful to Norman Comben for his continuing assistance over the last three years in developing these entries into their present form. He has also prepared the majority of the additional notes which are included where it is considered that these would be helpful. We are also grateful to the late Iain Pattison BSc FRCVS, for preparing the notes to items 356, 374, 647 and 648, to Jane Vincent for the note on Shepherd's Guides (561), to Robert L. Emory for providing the notes on the various issues of Stubbs (600), and to Victoria Smith for preparing the camera-ready copy.

Pauline Dingley
1992

Introduction

Until the end of the eighteenth century the diagnosis and treatment of the diseases and infirmities of animals was carried out predominantly by farriers – the shoeing smiths – and by a relatively smaller number of individuals, commonly regarded as of lesser intellect, who styled themselves cow doctors or cow leeches. The horse was then as important as the motor vehicle is today, and it is not surprising that a vast literature on farriery appeared during the seventeenth and eighteenth centuries. The word veterinary did not itself become established in this literature until the beginning of the nineteenth century, the first major works to be so titled being Delabere Blaine's *The outlines of the veterinary art* ..., 1802 (70) and Thomas Boardman's *Dictionary of the veterinary art* ..., 1802? and 1805(80).

Two important historical libraries collected and preserved the early farriery and veterinary literature during the nineteenth century, at the Royal Veterinary College in Camden Town, London, and at the Royal College of Veterinary Surgeons (the governing body of the veterinary profession), now in their Wellcome Library in Belgrave Square, London.

The Comben Collection complements the holdings of these two libraries. Its content of the scarce, early works on farriery published in the sixteenth to eighteenth centuries is particularly comprehensive. It also contains an important selection of the early more general titles on animal husbandry, most of which include significant passages on the diseases of animals and their treatments. While some duplication is inevitable, a number of scarce works are present which are not to be found in either the RVC or RCVS libraries.

The collection was formed over a period of 45 years from the early 1940s by Norman Comben BSc MRCVS, a veterinary surgeon fascinated by the origins of his profession. He was a founder member of the Veterinary History Society and its chairman for two years from 1973. He remains a member of the committee, and is actively involved with the production and distribution of the Society's bi-annual bulletin *Veterinary history*. He was awarded the J. T. Edwards Memorial Medal by The Royal College of Veterinary Surgeons in 1990 for outstanding work in the field of veterinary history.

The Comben Collection comprises some nine hundred printed books and pamphlets dating from the sixteenth to twentieth centuries, the majority predating 1850. There are 22 items from the sixteenth century, the earliest being the Aldine Press edition of Cato (et al.) *Libri de re rustica*, Venice, 1514 (555), 64 from the seventeenth, and nearly two hundred from the eighteenth century.

A great majority of the works are in English, and published in Britain, but some of the more important foreign books are also present – in particular the early Italian works on the horse such as Lorenzo Rusio's *Hippiatria*, Paris, 1532 (542); and Federigo Grisone's *Gli ordini di cavalcare*, 1550, 1561, and 1584 editions (302-304), noteworthy for its many woodcuts of horse bits.

Of the items of special interest, the apparently unique copy of *Snape's purging pill for horses* ..., 1692 (575) is important not only as the sole surviving copy of a second work by the author, Andrew Snape, of the well known *The anatomy of an horse* ..., 1683 (573), but also as the earliest recorded published catalogue of animal medicines for sale. There is a fine copy of Fitzherbert's *The boke of husbandry*, 1534 (261), the first book on agriculture printed in English. The works of Gervase Markham are particularly well represented; 25 examples include an exceptional copy of the scarce first edition of *Markhams maister-peece. Or, what doth a horse-man lacke* ..., 1610 (434). The collection abounds in such rarities, a number of which have been acquired from notable libraries such as those of the Earl of Kintore, and of Dr G. E. Fussell, the eminent agricultural historian.

Other rarities include John Halfpenny's *The gentleman's jocky*, London, 1671 (307), Matthew Allen's *The farrier's assistant*, London, 1737 (11), and John Bradstreet's *The farmers request*, Norwich, 1730 (103). The last is one of a number of rare provincial printings in the collection – others include Isaac Wyke's *The English and Welsh cattle doctor*, Abergavenny, ca.1812 (693) with parallel English and Welsh text, one of three Welsh items.

Among rare ephemera are a dozen advertising leaflets from the Victorian period and early twentieth century ranging from the Provincial Horse and Cattle Insurance Co.'s insurance against the cattle plague of 1865 (132), to White Horse's pocket booklet extolling the medicinal virtues of whisky for animals, 1912 (341). More substantial catalogues of veterinary equipment include Arnold & Sons, 7 editions, 1874 to 1905 (711-717) and Krohne & Sesemann, 1889 (780). Two early magazines are *The Farrier and naturalist*, the three published volumes, 1828-1830 (254), and *The Sportsman and veterinary recorder*, the 1835 volumes (592).

Fine illustrations include the *Maréchal* plates, 1769, from Diderot's *Encyclopédie* (223), George Stubbs's *The anatomy of the horse*, 1766 – the issue with plates watermarked 1823 (600); and Grisone's woodcuts mentioned above. Attractive, though less important, visual materials are the folded diagrams issued by Fores in 1848 (5 and 21), and the full set of foldout *Live stock models* first issued in 1914 by Vinton & Co. (14-20).

Among a number of sheep mark books, is the delightful hand-finished *Shepherd's guide; or a delineation of the wool and ear marks ... in Patterdale, Netherwasdale, Borrowdale* ..., 1819 (561). This is the first example of a local sheep mark guide. From the same period a little further north is James Hogg's *The shepherd's guide*, Edinburgh, 1807 (334), a fine copy in its original boards of one of the Scottish poet's less famous works.

Examination of the books in the collection reveals the quite astonishing extent to which texts were plagiarised by one author after another, sometimes down through more than a century. Perhaps this is not surprising, since of course no really significant advances in veterinary medicine were made until relatively recent times. Even veterinary anatomical plates were copied shamelessly, and the illustrations on pages 16 and 17 show how the original anatomical drawings first published by Ruini in 1598 were copied through two centuries until as late as 1806.

While a majority of the collection is of primary printed material it includes as back-up a substantial set of reference works and other secondary material – in particular bibliographies and catalogues of other collections, but also histories and biographies. A small collection of early works on poultry husbandry, formed by Norman Comben and acquired by the Science Museum Library in 1984, has now been integrated into the main Comben Collection.

References cited

Reference is made in notes in abbreviated form to certain standard works which are listed below. Where a copy of the work is in the Comben Collection the number of its catalogue entry is given.

Adams	Adams, H.M. Catalogue of books printed on the continent of Europe, 1501-1600 in Cambridge libraries. Cambridge: At the University Press, 1967. 2v.
Amery	Amery, G.D. The writings of Arthur Young. London: Royal Agricultural Society of England, 1925. (708)
BLC	The British Library general catalogue of printed books to 1975. London: Clive Bingley, 1979-1987. 360v.
Brunet	Brunet, J.C. Manuel du libraire et de l'amateur de livres. 5e éd. Paris: Firmin Didot, 1860-1865. 6v.
DNB	Dictionary of national biography. London: Smith, Elder, 1885-1901. 66v.
Fussell	Fussell, G.E. The old English farming books. London: Crosby Lockwood & Son: Pindar, 1947-1984. 4v. (747-751)
Huth	Huth, F.H. Works on horses and equitation. London: B. Quaritch, 1887. (771)
Mennessier de la Lance	Mennessier de la Lance, G.R. Essai de bibliographie hippique. Paris: L. Dorbon, 1915-1921. 3v. (788)
NUC pre-1956	The National union catalog pre-1956 imprints. London: Mansell, 1968-1981. 754v.
Perkins	Perkins, W.F. British and Irish writers on agriculture. 2nd ed. Lymington: Chas. T. King, 1932. (799)
Poynter	Poynter, F.N.L. A bibliography of Gervase Markham, 1568?-1637. Oxford: Oxford Bibliographical Society, 1962. (804)
Pugh	Pugh, L.P. From farriery to veterinary medicine, 1785-1795. Cambridge: W. Heffer and Son, 1962. (806)
RCVS	Royal College of Veterinary Surgeons. Library. Catalogue of the historical collection: books published before 1850. London: Royal College of Veterinary Surgeons, 1953. (817)
Rothamsted	Rothamsted Experimental Station. Library. Catalogue of the printed books on agriculture. [Harpenden: The Station, 1926.] (811) Library catalogue of printed books and pamphlets on agriculture. 2nd ed. Harpenden: The Station, 1940. (812)

RVC	Royal Veterinary College. Library. A catalogue of the books, pamphlets and periodicals up to 1850. London: Royal Veterinary College Library, 1965. (818)
Smith	Smith, Sir F. The early history of veterinary literature and its British development. London: Baillière, Tindall and Cox, 1919-1933. (Reprinted London: J.A. Allen & Co., 1976.) (823-830)
Southampton	University of Southampton. Library. Catalogue of the Walter Frank Perkins agricultural library. Southampton: The University Library, 1961. (846)
STC	Pollard, A.W. and Redgrave, G.R. A short-title catalogue of books printed in England, Scotland, & Ireland ... 1475-1640. 2nd ed. London: Bibliographical Society, 1986-1991. 3v.
Wellcome (pre-1641)	Wellcome Historical Medical Library. A catalogue of printed books. I. Books printed before 1641. London: Wellcome Historical Medical Library, 1962.
Wing	Wing, D. Short-title catalogue ... 1641-1700. 2nd ed. New York: Modern Language Association of America, 1972-1988. 3v.

Cataloguing conventions

The catalogue is arranged in two sections. The main collection of primary material forms the *Historic books* sequence and this is followed by the secondary material in the *Reference books* section.

Cataloguing is based on the Anglo-American cataloguing rules, second edition, 1988 revision (AACR 2) except for some typographical conventions.

In the description of the *Historic books* the mark of omission (...) is used to indicate omission of title page information from title, statement of responsibility and imprint. Full physical description is given including sequences of pages and leaves followed by the number of leaves or pages of plates. Unnumbered pages, etc. are indicated by the use of square brackets. Pagination is given for each volume in a multi-volume set. Illustrations are noted and the height of the book in centimetres is shown. The bibliographical format is also given for all books published up to 1850.

Notes in italics follow many entries. They include notes required to amplify the description, information about our particular copy and more discursive comments on points of interest. Cross-references to other items in the collection are given in parentheses.

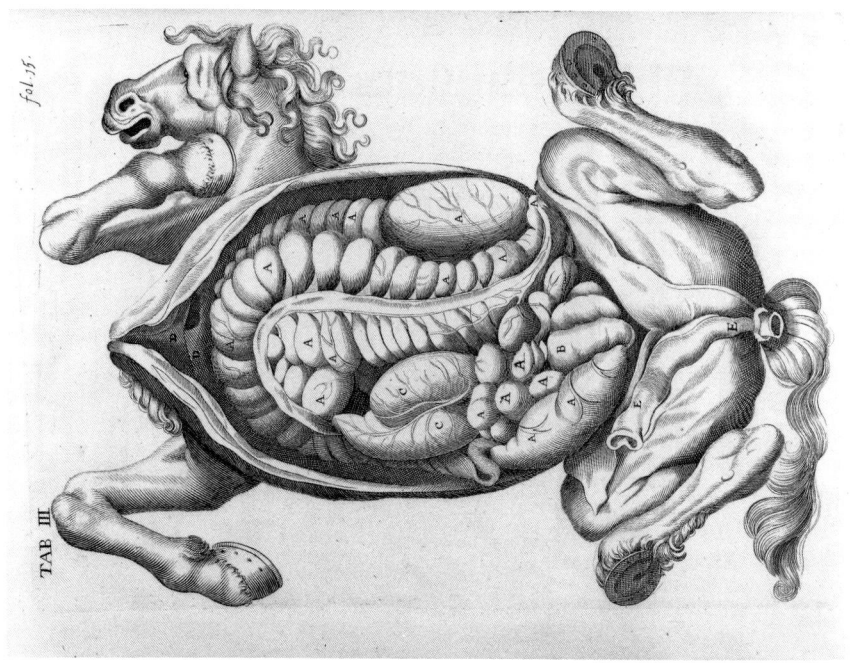

Snape 1683 (573)

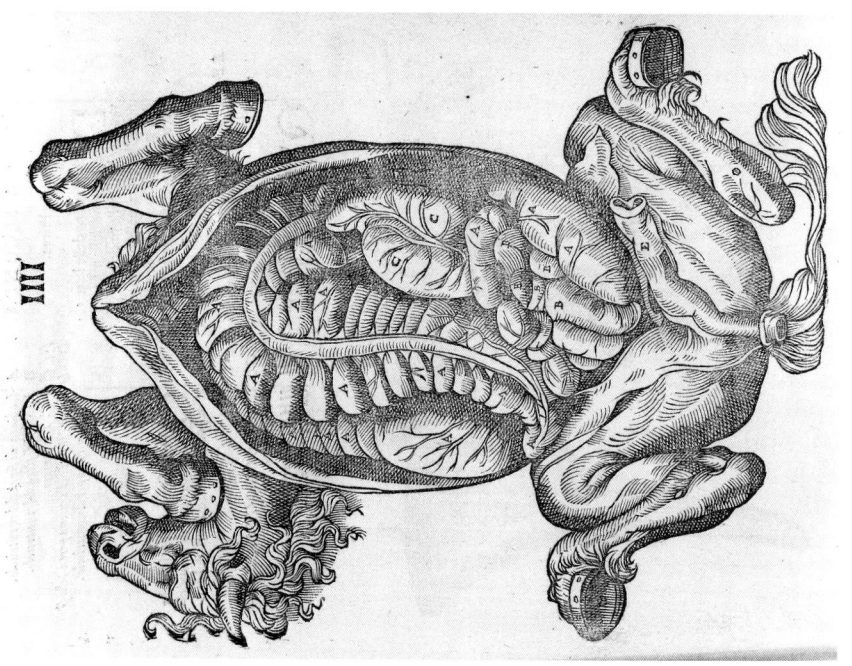

Ruini 1618 (541)

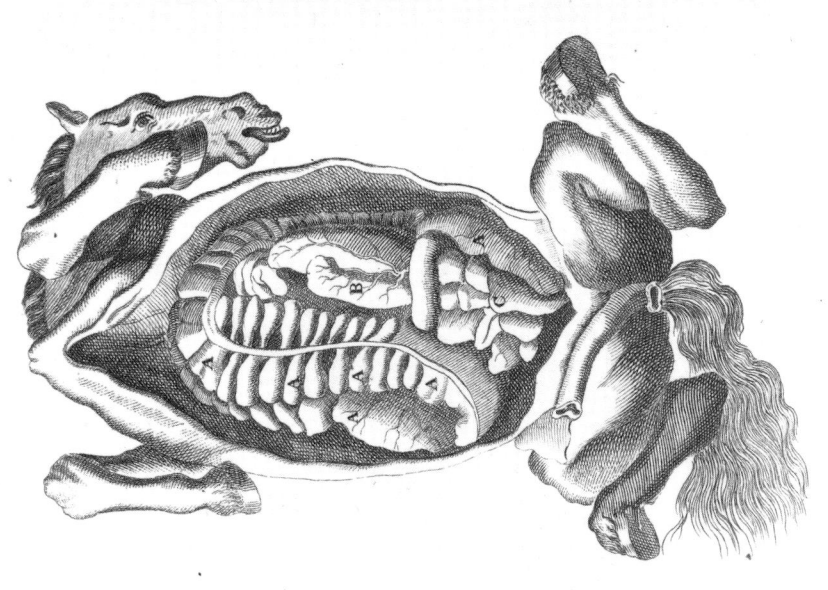

Burke 1806 (125)

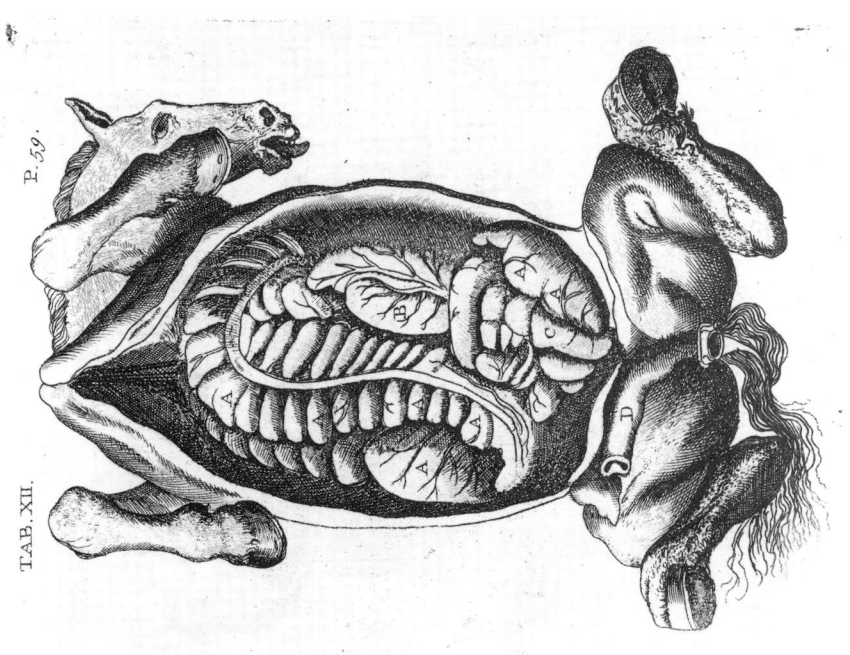

Gibson 1751 (289)

Plagiarism in veterinary anatomy, 1598-1806

Historic books

A.S.

1 The gentleman's compleat jockey: with the perfect horseman, and experienc'd farrier ... / by A.S. gent. — London: Printed for Henry Nelme ..., 1696. — [4], 168, [12]p, [1] folded leaf of plates: ill; 17cm (12mo)
Reference: Wing S4
Folded frontispiece repaired with some loss of text
Illustration: page 20

2 The gentleman's compleat jockey: with the perfect horse-man and experienc'd farrier ... / by A.S. gent. — London: Printed by T. Norris ... for Peter Parker ..., 1717. — 160, [8]p; 15cm (12mo)
Imperfect: plate missing, foot of some leaves cropped
*Much of the text is also found in the Conyers tract The compleat husbandman ... published under the name of G. Markham in 1707 (424) (Poynter *2.1.(a). and see note below re frontispiece plate)*

3 The husbandman, farmer, and grasier's compleat instructor : containing, choice and approved rules ... / by A.S. gent. — London: Printed for Henry Nelme ..., 1697. — [4], 168, [8]p, [1] folded leaf of plates: ill; 16cm (12mo)
Reference: Wing S7

4 The husbandman's instructor, or, Countryman's guide: containing plain and approved rules ... / by A.S. gent. — London: Printed, and sold by A. Conyers ..., [168-?]. — [4], 138, [2]p: ill; 15cm (12mo)
Preface signed: A.S. and J.L. (J. Lambert?)
The two titles by A.S. above have the same text, which is virtually identical to that of The country-man's treasure: ... by J. Lambert, gent. (373). The undated edition by A.S. has a crude wood-cut frontispiece plate depicting a bull, a sheep and a pig. The same frontispiece is found in The country-man's treasure: ... by Lambert (above) and in The compleat husbandman ... by G. Markham ..., 1707 (424); it is also found even more crudely re-drawn in The country-man's jewel: ... by M.S., gent, and others (415). The 1697 edition by A.S. has a different folded frontispiece; this copy is ex G.E. Fussell. The undated edition by A.S. is in an interesting early cloth binding
Illustration: page 21

5 The **AGES OF THE HORSE**: correctly exhibited by the tables of the teeth. — London: Fores, 1848. — 1 sheet: col.ill; 36x50cm folded to 13x11cm
Cover title
Mounted on linen. Between boards

AITON, William, 1760-1848

6 A treatise on the dairy breed of cows and dairy husbandry: with an account of the Lanarkshire breed of horses, &c. / by William Aiton. — Edinburgh: Bell & Bradfute, 1825. — [6], xviii, 195p, [4] leaves of plates: ill, port; 22cm (8vo)

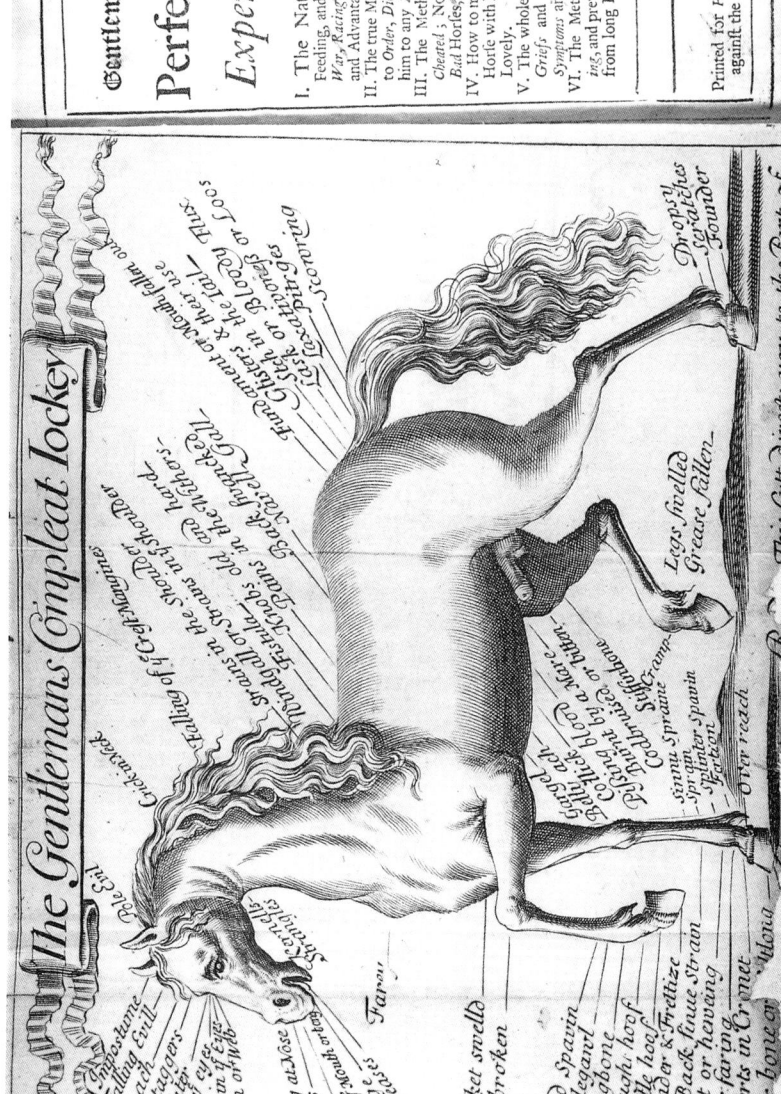

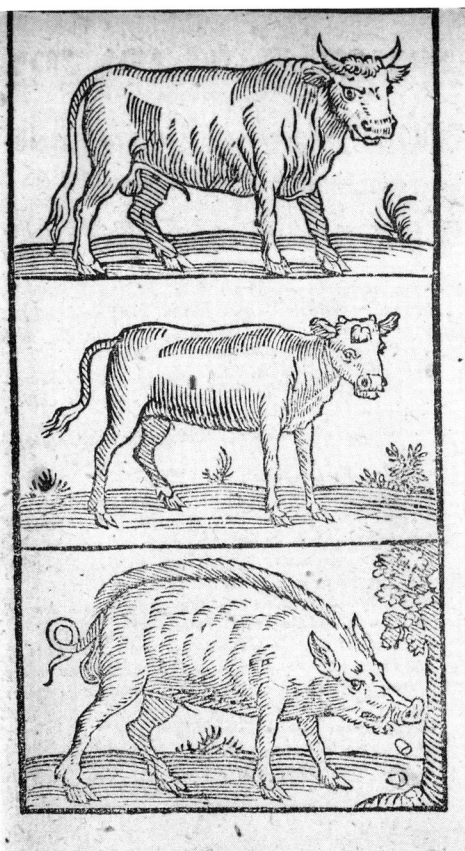

THE
Husbandman's Instructor,
OR,
Countryman's Guide.
CONTAINING

Plain and Approved RULES for the Ordering, Chusing, Breeding, Feeding, Buying, Selling, Fattening, and to Cure all manner of Diseases in

Bulls,	Swine,
Cows,	Goats,
Calves,	Asses,
Rams,	Mules,
Ewes,	Dogs,
Lambs,	Conies, &c.

To which is added,

Useful Directions for the right Ordering and Improving *POULTRY*; how to Cure their several Distempers, and make them very profitable to their Owners.

ALSO

Instructions for destroying all sorts of VERMIN, which infest *Houses, Fields, Granaries, Orchards, Gardens, Ships, Beds, Bedsteads,* or any other Places.

By *A. S.* Gent.

London printed, and sold by *A. Conyers* at the Ring in *Little-Britain.*   Pr. 1 s.

ALBERT VETERINARY COLLEGE

7 Rules and regulations of the Albert Veterinary College, Limited, Queen's Road, Bayswater. — London: A.H. Baily & Co., 1865. — [15]p; 21cm
Disbound
John Gamgee founded the New Veterinary College (or School) in Edinburgh in 1857; it was removed to London where it opened in the Queen's Road, Bayswater, as the Albert Veterinary College in 1865, but was closed down in 1868

ALBERTUS, Magnus, Saint, 1193?-1280

8 The secrets of Albertus Magnus: of the vertues of herbs, stones, and certain beasts ... — London: Printed by M.H. and T.M. and are to be sold by J. Wright [and 3 others], [1691?]. — [125]p; 15cm (8vo)
Signatures: A-H8
Bound with: Markham's method or epitome. — 11th ed. — London: W. Thackeray, 1684

ALDROVANDI, Ulisse, 1522-1605?

9 [Ornithologia. Vol.2, Book 14. English]
Aldrovandi on chickens: the Ornithology of Ulisse Aldrovandi (1600) Volume II, Book XIV / translated from the Latin with introduction, contents, and notes by L.R. Lind. — Norman: University of Oklahoma Press, c1963. — xxxvi, 447p: ill, port; 23cm

ALLEN, Lewis F. (Lewis Falley), 1800-1890

10 History of the short-horn cattle: their origin, progress and present condition / by Lewis F. Allen. — Buffalo, N.Y.: [L.F. Allen], 1878. — 266p, [10] leaves of plates: ill; 23cm

ALLEN, Matthew

11 The farrier's assistant: or, an essay on the nature and proceeding of distempers incident to horses ... / by Matthew Allen ... — London: Printed for Edward Symon, 1737. — [24], 144p; 19cm (8vo)
Not seen by Smith. Not in RVC or RCVS
Illustration: page 23

12 The **AMERICAN STANDARD OF PERFECTION**: as adopted by the American Poultry Association at its thirteenth annual meeting at Indianapolis, Indiana, 1888 containing a complete description of all the recognized varieties of fowls / edited by Harmon S. Babcock. — [S.l.]: The Association, 1891. — 244p; 18cm

13 The **AMERICAN STANDARD OF PERFECTION**: a complete description of all recognized varieties of fowls. As revised by the American Poultry Association at its thirty-fourth annual meeting at Niagara Falls ... and its thirty-fifth annual meeting at St. Louis, Missouri ... — [S.l]: The Association, 1910 (1912 printing). — 331p: ill.; 20cm

THE FARRIER's Assistant:

OR, AN ESSAY

ON THE

NATURE and PROCEEDING of DISTEMPERS

Incident to

HORSES.

VIZ.

I. Of Internal Diseases.

II. Of Visible and External Distempers.

III. Reasons why the FARSEY, Humours in the Eyes, and FEVERS, are more predominant this present Year 1736. than usual.

IV. A GENERAL REMEDY for most Distempers in Horses; it's Virtues, Manner of Operation, and how used and applied.

V. A Collection of CASES relating to the Distempers here treated of.

By MATTHEW ALLEN,

FARRIER, in *Coleman-street*.

LONDON,

Printed for EDWARD SYMON, against the *Royal Exchange*. MDCCXXXVII.

14 **ANATOMICAL MODEL OF THE BULL**: five coloured plates (with key). — 2nd ed. — London: Vinton & Co., [192-]. — [4], 4p: multi-layered model; 19x26cm. — (Vinton's live stock models; no.3)

15 **ANATOMICAL MODEL OF THE COW**: five coloured plates (with key). — 3rd ed. — London: Vinton & Co., [192-]. — [4], 4p: multi-layered model; 19x26cm. — (Vinton's live stock models; no.4)

16 **ANATOMICAL MODEL OF THE HEN**: five coloured plates (with key). — London: Vinton & Co., [192-]. — [4], 4p: multi-layered model; 19x26cm. — (Vinton's live stock models; no.7)

17 **ANATOMICAL MODEL OF THE HORSE**: five coloured plates (with key). — 2nd ed. — London: Vinton & Co., [192-]. — [4], 4p: multi-layered model; 19x26cm. — (Vinton's live stock models; no.1)

18 **ANATOMICAL MODEL OF THE MARE**: five coloured plates (with key). — 2nd ed. — London: Vinton & Co., [192-]. — [4], 4p: multi-layered model; 19x26cm. — (Vinton's live stock models; no.2)

19 **ANATOMICAL MODEL OF THE PIG**: five coloured plates (with key). — London: Vinton & Co., [1914]. — [7]p: multi-layered model; 19x26cm. — (Vinton's live stock models; no.6)

20 **ANATOMICAL MODEL OF THE SHEEP**: five coloured plates (with key). — London: Vinton & Co., [1914]. — [7]p: multi-layered model; 19x26cm. — (Vinton's live stock models; no.5)

21 The **ANATOMY OF THE HORSE'S FOOT**: representing the blood vessels, ligaments, bones ... — London: Fores, 1848. — 1 sheet: col.ill; 36x50cm folded to 13x11cm
Cover title
Mounted on linen. Between boards

ARMATAGE, George
22 The thermometer as an aid to diagnosis in veterinary medicine / by George Armatage. — 3rd ed. rev. and enl. — London: F. Warne and Co., 1894. — 71p: ill; 18cm

ASH, Edward C., b.1888
23 Poultry (light breeds): and how to know them / by Edward C. Ash. — London: Epworth Press, [1922]. — 62, [2]p: ill; 19cm

ASTLEY, Philip, 1742-1814

24 Astley's projects, in his management of the horse: rendering it calm on the road, in harness, &c. ... being an abridgement of his popular and most valuable book of Equestrian education ... — London: Printed by T. Burton ... sold by S. Creed ..., 1804. — xv, [1], 72p, [1] folded leaf of plates: ill; 17cm (8vo)

25 Astley's system of equestrian education: exhibiting the beauties and defects of the horse ... — [London]: Sold by C. Creed ..., 1801. — vi, [7]-192, [14]p, [10] leaves of plates: ill, port.; 22cm (8vo)
Errata: last p.
Imperfect: plate facing p.183 missing

26 Astley's system of equestrian education: exhibiting the beauties and defects of the horse ... — The fifth edition. — London: Printed by T. Burton ... sold by S. Creed ..., [1801?]. — xvi, 197, [3]p, [10] leaves of plates: ill, port.; 23cm (8vo)

B., J.
see BLAGRAVE, Joseph, 1610-1682

B., N.
The farrier's and horseman's dictionary
see N.B.

BAILY, John

27 Fowls: a plain and familiar treatise on the principal breeds, with which is reprinted the third edition of The Dorking fowl: hints for its management and feeding for the table / by John Baily. — London: Henningham and Hollis, 1852. — xi, 58, [2]p; 16cm

BAKEWELL, Robert, 1768-1843

28 Observations on the influence of soil and climate upon wool: from which is deduced a certain and easy method of improving the quality of English clothing wools ... / by Robert Bakewell; with occasional notes and remarks by the Right Hon. Lord Somerville. — London: Printed for J. Harding ..., 1808. — ix, [1], 157p; 21cm (8vo)
Errata: on p.[x]

BARET, Michael

29 An hipponomie or The vineyard of horsemanship: deuided into three bookes ... / by Michaell Baret, practitioner and professor of the same art. — London: Printed by George Eld, 1618. — [20], 122, [20], 139, [13], 101, [1], 23, [2]p; 19cm (8vo)
The 3 pts. have separate title pages and pagination
Reference: STC 1412
Illustration: page 26

AN HIPPONOMIE OR THE VINEYARD OF HORSEMANSHIP:

Deuided into three Bookes.

1. The Theorick Part, intreating of the inward Knowledge of the Man.
2. The first Practicke Part, shewing how to worke according to that Knowledge.
3. The second Practicke Part, declaring how to apply both hunting and running Horses to the true grounds of this Art.

In which is plainly laid open the Art of Breeding, Riding, Training and Dieting of the said Horses.

Wherein also many errors in this Art, heretofore published, are manifestly detected.

By MICHAELL BARET, *Practitioner and Professor of the same Art.*

LONDON,
Printed by GEORGE ELD. 1618.

BARET, René

30 La marechallerie françoise, où le traitté de la connoissance des cheuaux: du iugement et remede de leur maladie / par René Baret ... — Troisiesme edition augmente'e. — A Paris: Chez Sebastien Piquet ..., 1654. — [8], 105, [2]p: ill; 22cm (4to)
Added engraved t.p. dated 1651 is pasted on inserted leaf
Reference: Mennessier de la Lance v.1, p.71
Not known to Huth. Ex J.H. Anderhub in his typical vellum binding with slip case, but not the copy listed in the sale of his library by Karl & Faber in Munich in 1963

BARLOW, Henry

31 The cattle keeper's guide, or complete directory, for the choice and management of cattle: whether horses, oxen, cows ... / by Henry Barlow ... — London: William Darton, jun. ..., 1819. — iv, 68p, [1] folded leaf of plates: ill; 18cm (12mo)
Plagiarised from J. Ringsted, The cattle-keeper's assistant

32 The cattle keeper's guide: or, complete directory for the choice and management of cattle, whether horses, oxen, cows ... / by Henry Barlow. — Halifax: Milner and Sowerby, 1863. — xiii, 7-84, 4p, [1] leaf of plates: ill; 16cm
Last 4p. are advertisements
Plagiarised from J. Ringsted, The cattle-keeper's assistant
Not known to Smith or to Fussell. Not in RVC or RCVS

BARLOW, J. H.

33 The art and method of hatching and rearing all kinds of domestic poultry and game birds by steam: also is added the method by which the Egyptians hatch ninety-six millions a year / invented by J.H. Barlow. — London: J.H. Barlow, 1827. — 20p, [4] leaves of plates (1 folded); 22cm (8vo)

34 The daily progress and extraordinary appearance of the chick in the egg, and the changes which take place during hatching in the steam apparatus / invented by J.H. Barlow. — London: J.H. Barlow, 1824. — [32]p, [2] leaves of plates (1 folded): ill; 20cm (8vo)

BARTLET, J. (John), 1716?-1772

35 The gentleman's farriery: or, a practical treatise on the diseases of horses: wherein the best writers on that subject have been consulted ... / by J. Bartlet. — The second edition improved. — London: Printed for John Nourse ... and Joseph Pote, at Eton, 1754. — [2], xxiv, 357, [11]p, [3] leaves of plates (1 folded): ill; 18cm (8vo)
Errata: on p.[9]
Horizontal chain lines

36 The gentleman's farriery: or, a practical treatise on the diseases of horses: wherein the best writers on that subject have been consulted ... / by J. Bartlet. — The ninth edition, revised. — London: Printed for J. Nourse ... [and 8 others], 1777. — xxviii, 370, [10]p, [6] leaves of plates (4 folded): ill; 19cm (8vo)
Horizontal chain lines
Illustration: page 29

37 The gentleman's farriery; or, a practical treatise on the diseases of horses: wherein the best writers on that subject have been consulted ... / by J. Bartlet. — The twelfth edition, revised. — London: Printed for C. Nourse ... [and 6 others], 1788. — xxviii, 370, [10]p, [6] leaves of plates (4 folded): ill; 18cm (8vo)
Horizontal chain lines
Pages xxv-xxviii misbound between p.[4] and [5]

38 The gentleman's farriery; or, a practical treatise on the diseases of horses: wherein the best writers on that subject have been consulted ... / by J. Bartlet. — The twelfth edition revised. — London: Printed for A. Millar, W. Law, and R. Cater; and for Wilson, Spence, and Mawman, York, 1796. — xxiii, [1] (blank), [13]-252p, VI leaves of plates (4 folded) : ill; 18cm (12mo)
The 2nd edition (1754) has a half-title; frontispiece vignette of a horse wearing a blanket in a stable; folded plate, "... of the two heads and trepan" at p.348; and a plate of the "nicking machine" at p.354. The later editions do not have half-titles. The 9th (1777) and 12th (1788) editions have the same frontispiece and plates as above, and three additional folded plates of Anatomy (of the hoof) at the end of the book. The "12th edition revised" (1796) has again the same plates, but the three folded Anatomy plates have been re-drawn and are bound in throughout the text

39 Pharmacopoeia hippiatrica: or, the gentleman farrier's repository: of elegant and approved remedies for the diseases of horses; in two books ... / by J. Bartlet ... — Eton: Printed by J. Pote for T. Pote, 1764. — xii, 382, [1]p; 18cm (8vo)
Errata: last p.

40 Pharmacopoeia hippiatrica: or, the gentleman farrier's repository: of elegant and approved remedies for the diseases of horses; in two books ... / by J. Bartlet ... — The second edition. — Eton: Printed for T. Pote, 1766. — xiv, 394 [i.e.402]p; 18cm (8vo)
Some ms notes

BARTLEY, Nehemiah

41 A series of letters: on the national importance, as well as the individual benefit, of extending the growth of fine clothing wool, by interbreeding with Spanish rams and British ewes ... / by Nehemiah Bartley ... — Bath: Printed by W. Meyler, and sold by G. and J. Robinson, London ..., 1804. — iv, [5]-84p; 22cm (8vo)
Disbound

BEAUMONT, T.

42 The complete cow doctor: being a treatise on the disorders incident to horned cattle ... / by T. Beamont [sic] ... — Leeds: Printed by George Wilson ..., 1812. — 108p; 17cm (12mo)

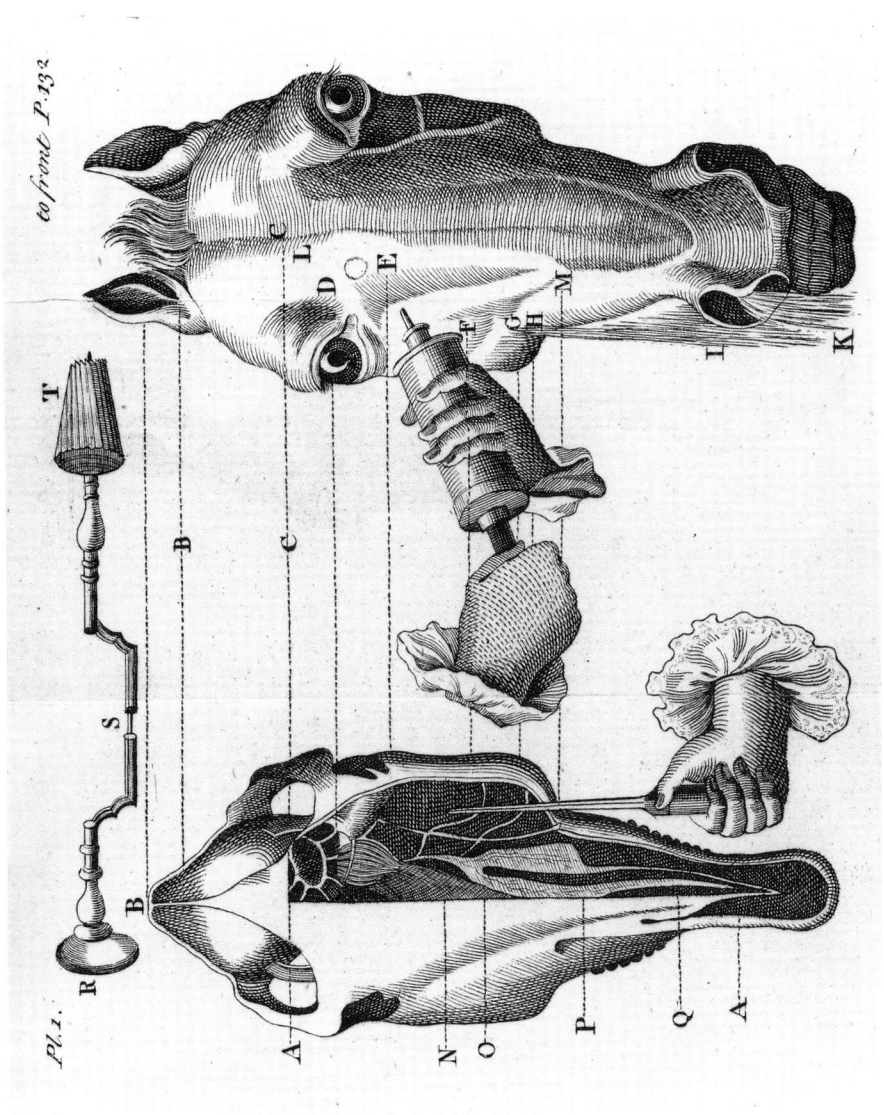

43 The complete cow doctor: being a treatise on the disorders incident to horned cattle ... / by T. Beaumont. — Halifax: Milner and Sowerby, 1863. — 92, 4p, [1] leaf of plates: ill; 16cm

44 The complete new cow doctor: being a treatise on the disorders incident to horned cattle ... to which is added, a concise treatise on farriery ... / by T. Beaumont. — New ed. improved. — Manchester: Printed by S. Johnson, 1835. — 140, [4]p; 15cm
The complete farrier has separate t.p.
Not known to Smith or to Fussell. In the edition of 1812 the author's name is given as BEAMONT. The edition of 1835 is of interest as being printed in gatherings of 9 leaves

BEETON, Samuel Orchart, 1831-1877
45 Beeton's book of poultry and domestic animals: showing how to rear and manage them in sickness and in health. — London: Ward, Lock, [1870]. — xii, p.353-832, [20]p, [2] leaves of plates: ill (some col.); 19cm
Reissue of part of The book of home pets
Advertisements on [20]p at end

46 Beeton's poultry book: containing a clear account of the best modes of producing eggs, and rearing chickens, ducks, geese, and turkeys, so as to combine a pleasant occupation with profitable investment. — 2nd ed. — London: Ward, Lock & Tyler, [187-]. — 48p; 14cm
Part of Beeton's penny books

BELLAMY, T.
47 Medicines for the cure of the diseases incident to cattle, sheep, etc.: particularly an infallible remedy for the scouring in beasts / by T. Bellamy. — 9th ed. — Bristol: Printed by Philip Rose, jun., 1841. — 40p; 22cm (4to)
Subscribers' names: p.[24]-37
Half title: Recipes to prepare and administer various medicines for the cure ...
Bound with: High farming / by James Caird. — 5th ed. — Edinburgh: W. Blackwood and Sons, 1849

48 Recipes to prepare and administer various medicines for the cure of the diseases incident to cattle, sheep, &c.: particularly an infallible remedy for the scouring in beasts / by T. Bellamy. — Bath: Printed by W. Meyler, 1804. — viii, [9]-30p; 21cm (8vo)
Subscribers' names: p.19-25
Imperfect: first 2 prelim. leaves missing. Description from NUC pre-1956, v.45, p.104. Ms. note laid in
Not known to Smith. Not in RVC or RCVS

BEMENT, C. N. (Caleb N.), 1791?-1868

49 The American poulterer's companion: a practical treatise on the breeding, rearing, fattening, and general management of the various species of domestic poultry / by C.N. Bement. — 5th ed. — New York: Harper & Brothers, 1847. — [6], 379p: ill.; 20cm (12mo)

50 The American poulterer's companion: a practical treatise on the breeding, rearing, and general management of various species of domestic poultry / by C.N. Bement. — New ed., enl. and improved. — New York: Harper & Brothers, 1856. — 304p, [19] leaves of plates: ill; 20cm
Lacks plate facing p.104

BENNETT, John C.

51 The poultry book: a treatise on breeding and general management of domestic fowls ... / by John C. Bennett. — Boston: Phillips, Sampson, 1851. — 310, [9]p: ill; 20cm
Advertisements on [9]p at end

BENNETT, Richard, 1844-1900

52 History of corn milling / by Richard Bennett and John Elton. Vol.1: Handstones, slave & cattle mills. — London: Simpkin, Marshall and Co., 1898. — xix, 246p, [1] leaf of plates: ill, facsim.; 22cm

53 History of corn milling / by Richard Bennett and John Elton. Vol.2: Watermills and windmills. — London: Simpkin, Marshall and Co., 1899. — xvi, 343p: ill; 22cm

54 History of corn milling / by Richard Bennett and John Elton. Vol.3: Feudal laws and customs. — London: Simpkin, Marshall and Co., 1900. — xii, 330p, [4] folded leaves of plates: ill; 22cm

55 History of corn milling / by Richard Bennett and John Elton. Vol.4: Some feudal mills: with memoir of the late Richard Bennett / by John Elton. — London: Simpkin, Marshall and Co., 1904. — xvi, 226p: ill, port.; 22cm

BERNERS, Juliana
The book of St Albans
see BOOK OF ST ALBANS

BERRY, Henry

56 Improved short-horns: and their pretensions stated ... / Henry Berry. — 2nd ed. — London: James Ridgway, 1830. — 81p; 22cm (4to)
Disbound

57 Prize essay, on the breeding & management of cattle: and the most approved system of farming ... / written for and presented to the Liverpool Agricultural Society by the Rev. Henry Berry; also, a letter, containing a remedy for fog sickness, hoven, or blown ... by Richard Sumner. — Liverpool: J.F. Cannell, 1831. — 16p; 21cm (4to)
Disbound

BIGGLE, Jacob

58 Biggle poultry book: a concise and practical treatise on the management of farm poultry / by Jacob Biggle. — Philadelphia: Wilmer Atkinson, 1895. — 160p: ill. (some col.); 14cm. — (Biggle farm library; no.3)

59 Biggle poultry book: a concise and practical treatise on the management of farm poultry / by Jacob Biggle. — 7th ed. — Philadelphia: Wilmer Atkinson, 1909. — 162p: ill. (some col.); 14cm. — (Biggle farm library)

60 The **BLACKFACE SHEEP KEEPERS' GUIDE**: for the north-eastern moors of Yorkshire ... also, a list of sheep marks with the names of the owners. — [S.l.]: Blackface Sheep Breeders' Association, 1924. — 63p: ill, ports; 19cm
Newspaper cuttings, photographs, and ms notes laid in

BLACKLOCK, Ambrose, 1816-1873
61 A treatise on sheep: the best means for their improvement ... / by Ambrose Blacklock. — 12th ed. — London: Groombridge & Sons, 1853. — xiii, 236p, [2], VIII leaves of plates: ill(some col.); 15cm
Two copies of plate I bound in

BLAGRAVE, Joseph, 1610-1682
62 The epitome of the art of husbandry: comprising all necessary directions for the improvement of it ... / by J.B. gent. — London: Printed for Ben. Billingsley and Obadiah Blagrave ..., 1669. — [16], 306, [6]p, [1] leaf of plates: ill; 15cm (8vo)
Last [6]p are advertisements
Reference: Wing (2nd ed.) B3115
T.p. repaired

63 The epitomie of the art of husbandry: comprizing all necessary directions for the improvement of it ... to which is annexed by way of appendix, a new method ... / by J.B. gent. — London: Printed for Benjamin Billingsley ..., 1685. — [7], 246, 136, [8]p, [2] leaves of plates: ill; 17cm (8vo)
New additions to the art of husbandry has separate t.p., additional engraved t.p. and separate pagination

BLAINE, Delabere, 1770-1845
64 Canine pathology, or a full description of the diseases of dogs: with their causes, symptoms, and mode of cure ... / by Delabere Blaine ... — London: Printed for T. Boosey ..., 1817. — [6], 1, 184, [2]p; 22cm (8vo)

65 Canine pathology; or, a description of the diseases of dogs: with their causes, symptoms, and mode of cure ... / Delabere Blaine. — 2nd ed. — London: Boosey and Sons, 1824. — x, [7]-326p; 22cm (8vo)

66 A concise description of the distemper in dogs: with an account of the discovery of an efficacious remedy for it / by Delabere Blaine ... — Fourth edition, with great additions. To which is added The outlines of a plan for a general arrangement and distribution of remedies for the prevalent diseases of the horse and dog. — London: Printed for and sold by T. Boosey ... and by the venders of the Medicinal Powder, 1806. — [4], 73, [3]p, [1] leaf of plates: ill; 17cm (12mo)
The outlines of a plan has separate t.p.
Illustration: page 34

67 A domestic treatise on the diseases of horses and dogs: so conducted as to enable persons to practice with ease and success on their own animals ... / by Delabere Blaine ... — London: Printed for T. Boosey ..., 1803. — [2], 179, [3]p, [1] leaf of plates: ill; 18cm (12mo)

68 A domestic treatise on the diseases of horses and dogs: so conducted as to enable persons to practice with ease and success on their own animals ... / Delabere Blaine ... — Second edition. — London: Printed for T. Boosey ..., 1803. — [2], 204, [4]p, [1] leaf of plates: ill; 19cm (12mo)

69 A domestic treatise on the diseases of horses and dogs: so conducted as to enable persons to practise with ease and success on their own animals ... / by Delabere Blaine. — Fourth edition, with very large additions. — London: Printed for T. Boosey ..., 1810. — [2], iii, [4]-249, [11]p; 20cm (12mo)

70 The outlines of the veterinary art; or, the principles of medicine: as applied to a knowledge of the structure, functions, and oeconomy of the horse, the ox, the sheep, and the dog ... / by Delabere Blaine ... — London: Printed by A. Strahan ... for T.N. Longman and O. Rees ... and T. Boosey ..., 1802. — 2v (xxii, [2], 560p, [2] leaves of plates (one folded);viii, 783, [1]p, 3-9 leaves of plates (5 folded)): ill; 22cm (8vo)
Provenance: Earl of Kintore (armorial bookplate)
In this copy, v.2 p.403-406 (Dd 2,3) and 407-408 (Dd 4) (Contents for Part III) are misbound with the prelims. There appear to be no p.409-416, and only 4 leaves in gathering Dd although the book is otherwise octavo. The catchword from Dd 4 (verso) to Ee 1 is correct, and the listing of Contents is complete

71 The outlines of the veterinary art; or, the principles of medicine: as applied to the structure, functions, and oeconomy, of the horse ... / by Delabere Blaine ... — The second edition, entirely recomposed, with numerous alterations, important additions, and new plates. — London: Printed for T. Boosey [and 3 others], [1816]. — [iii]-xvi, xii [i.e.xiii], [1] (blank), 663, [3]p, 9 leaves of plates (some folded): ill; 22cm (8vo)
2p. advertisement for R. Long, veterinary instrument maker, at rear

A CONCISE DESCRIPTION
OF THE
DISTEMPER IN DOGS:
WITH AN ACCOUNT OF THE DISCOVERY
OF
AN EFFICACIOUS REMEDY FOR IT.

Fourth Edition, with great Additions.

TO WHICH IS ADDED,

The Outlines of a Plan

For a general Arrangement and Distribution of Remedies for the prevalent Diseases of the Horse and Dog.

BY DELABERE BLAINE,
Veterinary Surgeon.

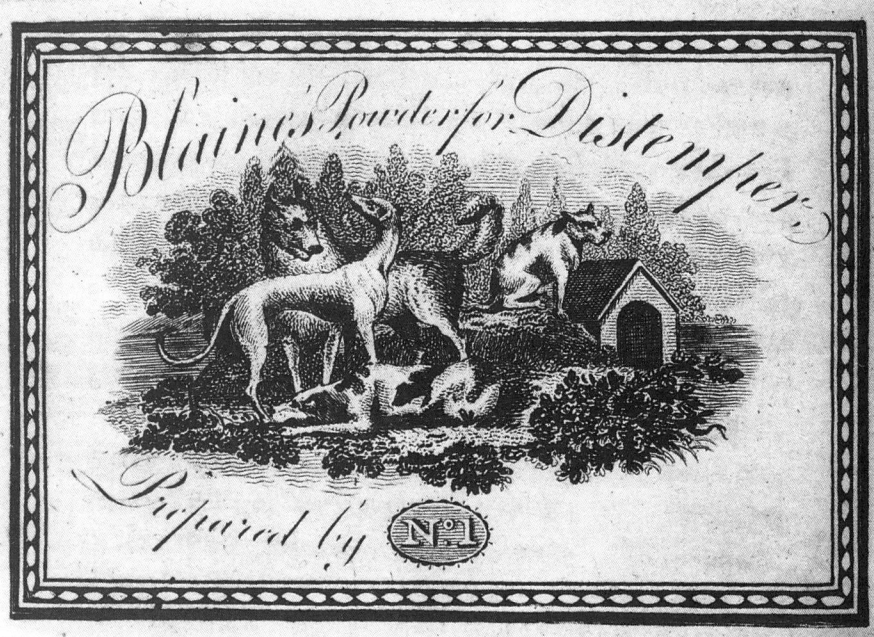

LONDON:
PRINTED FOR AND SOLD BY T. BOOSEY, 4, OLD BROAD STREET,
And by the Venders of the Medicinal Powder.
1806.

BLAINE, Ephraim
72 The village farrier: a plain and familiar treatise on the various disorders incident to the horse ... / by Ephraim Blaine. — 2nd ed. — London: Printed for the author, and sold by Thomas Tegg, 1831. — [2], ii, 228p; 19cm (12mo)

BLAIR, Mrs Fergusson, 1822-1904
73 The henwife: her own experience in her own poultry-yard / by Mrs Fergusson Blair; coloured illustrations by Harrison Weir. — Edinburgh: Thomas C. Jack; London: Hamilton, Adams and Co., 1861. — [10], xi, 192, [1]p, [8] leaves of plates: ill (chiefly col.) ; 17cm

74 The henwife: her own experience in her own poultry-yard / by Mrs Fergusson Blair; coloured illustrations by Harrison Weir. — 2nd ed. — Edinburgh: Thomas C. Jack; London: Hamilton, Adams, and Co., 1861. — 218p, [10] leaves of plates: ill (chiefly col.); 18cm
Decorated full red morocco binding, with brass clasp

75 The henwife: her own experience in her own poultry-yard / by Mrs Fergusson Blair; with illustrations by Harrison Weir. — 5th ed. — Edinburgh: Inglis & Jack, 1865. — 216p, [10] leaves of plates: ill (chiefly col.); 17cm

BLUNDEVILLE, Thomas, d.1605
76 The foure chiefest offices belonging to horsemanship: that is to saie, the office of the breeder, of the rider, of the keeper, and of the ferrer ... / by Thomas Blundeuill of Newton Flotman in Norffolke. — Imprinted at London: By Henrie Denham ..., 1580. — [6], 22, [7], 81, [3], 22, [5], 86 leaves: ill; 19cm (4to)
Parts have separate title pages and foliation. Part 2: The art of riding, is rev. and abridged translation of: F. Grisone, Ordini di cavalcare
Reference: STC3154
Imperfect: t.p. and 2nd leaf torn

77 The foure chiefest offices belonging to horsemanship: that is to say, the office of the breeder, of the rider, of the keeper, and of the ferrer ... / by Master Blundeuill of Newton Flotman in Norffolke. — Imprinted at London: by Humfrey Lownes, for the Company of the Stationers, 1609. — [6], 22, [7], 81, [3], 22, [5], 86 leaves: ill; 19cm (4to)
Parts have separate title pages and foliation. Part 2 is rev. and abridged translation of: F. Grisone, Ordini di cavalcare
Reference: STC3157
Imperfect: t.p. and last leaf missing. Description from NUC pre-1956, v.62, p.183

BLUNT, John
78 Practical farriery; or, the complete directory: in whatever relates to the food, management, and cure of diseases incident to horses / by John Blunt ... — London: Printed for G. Robinson ..., 1773. — viii, 316, [8]p, III leaves of plates (1 folded): ill; 17cm (12mo)

79 Practical farriery; or, the complete directory: in whatever relates to the food, management, and cure of diseases incident to horses / by John Blount [sic] ... — The second edition. — London: Printed for G. Robinson ..., 1779. — viii, 316, [8]p, III leaves of plates (1 folded): ill; 18cm (12mo)

BOARDMAN, Thomas
80 A dictionary of the veterinary art: containing all the modern improvements ... / by Thomas Boardman ... — London: Printed for George Kearsley ... by T. Davison ..., 1805. — vii, [871]p, XXIX [i.e.39] leaves of plates: ill; 28cm (4to)
Errors: p.[3]
Printed in columns
The first encyclopaedic work to use the word Veterinary in the title, in contrast to the various Dictionaries of farriery, and similar, published previously

BOLTON, John
81 John Bolton's remarks on pleuro pneumonia; or lung distemper in cattle. — Dublin: F.H. Judge, 1854. — 4p; 23cm

[The BOOK OF ST ALBANS]
82 The gentlemans academie. Or, the booke of S. Albans: containing three most exact and excellent bookes: the first of hawking, the second of all proper termes of hunting, and the last of armorie / all compiled by Iuliana Barnes ...; and now reduced into a better method, by G.M. — London: Printed for Humfrey Lownes ..., 1595. — [4], 95 leaves: ill, coats of arms; 20cm (4to)
G.M. is Gervase Markham
Reference: STC (2nd ed.) 3314
Some ms notes

83 The boke of Saint Albans: containing treatises on hawking, hunting, and cote armour: printed at Saint Albans by the Schoolmaster-printer in 1486 reproduced in facsimile / by Dame Juliana Berners; with an introduction by William Blades. — London: Elliot Stock, 1881. — 32, [177]p: ill, coats of arms, facsims; 29cm

84 English hawking and hunting in The boke of St Albans: a facsimile edition of sigs a2-f8 of The boke of St Albans (1486) / [edited] by Rachel Hands. — London: Oxford University Press, 1975. — lxix, 195p: col facsims; 23cm. — (Oxford English monographs)

BOOTHBY, Richard
85 A treatise on the diseases of cattle: with the mode of cure ... / by Richard Boothby, of Doncaster. — Doncaster: Printed by W. Sheardown ..., 1808. — [6], 58, [1]p; 23cm (8vo)
Subscribers names: p.1-4

BOSWELL, George

86 A treatise on watering meadows: wherein are shewn some of the many advantages ... — Third edition, with many additions. — Dublin: Printed by J. Moore ..., 1792. — viii, 120p, [5] folded leaves of plates: ill, plans; 22cm (8vo)
By George Boswell
Bound with: Facts and observations relative to sheep, wool, ploughs, and oxen / by John, Lord Somerville. — London: W. Miller, 1803

BOSWELL, Peter

87 The poultry-yard: a practical view of the best method of selecting, rearing and breeding the various species of domestic fowl / by Peter Boswell. — New ed. — London: Routledge, 1845. — x, 200p; 15cm (12mo)

BOUTROLLE, J. G.

88 Le parfait bouvier, ou instruction concernant la connoissance des boeufs & vaches ... On y a joint deux petits traités pour les moutons & porcs; ainsi que plusieurs remèdes pour les chevaux ... / par M. J.G. Boutrolle. — A Rouen: Chez la veuve Besongne ..., 1766. — [2], iii, [2] (blank)-135, [1] (blank), 1-70, [5], [1-2] (blank)p; 17cm (12mo)
"Dissertation sur la maladie des chevaux qu'on nomme la morve" is separately paginated

BOWES, James L.

89 The sheep-rot / by James L. Bowes. — London: Henry Sotheran and Co., 1880. — 39p, [2] folded leaves of plates: ill, maps; 23cm

BOWMAN, W.

90 The complete cow doctor, and farrier: describing the symptoms of the disorders ... / by W. Bowman. — London: Baldwin and Cradock, 1830. — 84, [89]-122p; 18cm (12mo)
The complete farrier has separate t.p.
Not known to Smith. Not in RVC or RCVS

BRACKEN, Henry, 1697-1764

91 Farriery improved: or, a compleat treatise upon the art of farriery: wherein is fully explain'd the nature, structure, and mechanism of that noble and useful creature a horse ... / by Henry Bracken ... — London: Printed for J. Clarke ... and J. Shuckburgh ..., 1737. — xvi, [8], 616, [26]p; 20cm (8vo)
Subscribers names: p.[1-8] (2nd group)

92 Farriery improved: or, a compleat treatise upon the art of farriery: wherein is fully explain'd the nature, structure, and mechanism of that noble and useful creature a horse ... / by Henry Bracken ... — Dublin: Printed by R. Reilly for G. Ewing ..., 1737. — xv, [1], 382, [26]p; 21cm (8vo)

93 Farriery improv'd: or, a compleat treatise upon the art of farriery: wherein is fully explain'd, the nature, structure, and mechanism of that noble and useful creature, a horse ... / by Henry Bracken ... — The second edition. — London: Printed for J. Clarke ... and J. Shuckburgh ..., 1739. — viii, [2], 363, [35]p; 17cm (12mo)

94 Farriery improv'd: or, a compleat treatise upon the art of farriery: wherein is fully explained the nature, structure, and mechanism of that noble and useful creature, a horse ... Vol.II / by Henry Bracken ... — London: Printed for J. Hodges ..., 1740. — xvi, 277, [29]p; 17cm (12mo)

95 Farriery improv'd: or, a compleat treatise upon the art of farriery: wherein is fully explain'd the nature, structure and mechanism of that noble and useful creature, a horse ... / by Henry Bracken ... — The eighth edition. — London: Printed for J. Shuckburgh ...; and W. Johnston ..., 1756. — viii, [2], 363, [35]p; 17cm (12mo)
Ms. notes

96 Farriery improv'd: or, a compleat treatise upon the art of farriery: wherein is fully explained the nature, structure, and mechanism of that noble and useful creature, a horse ... Vol.II / by Henry Bracken ... — The sixth edition, with large additions. — London: Printed for J. Hodges ..., 1757. — xvi, 298, [22]p; 17cm (12mo)
Ms. notes
Bracken's Farriery improved ... was first published in both London and Dublin in 1737 as a single 8vo volume. Although editions continued to be published in 8vo in Dublin, all subsequent London editions were in smaller 12mo format. A supplement was published in 1740 as Volume II; dates and editions in 2-volume sets are consequently always at variance. All London 12mo editions of the second volume (only) have half-titles

97 Farriery improved; or, a complete treatise on the art of farriery: wherein is fully explained the nature and structure of that useful creature, a horse ... / by Henry Bracken ... — Second edition. — London: Printed by W. Cooper for Nathaniel Frobisher ... York, 1789. — iv, 142p, [8] folded leaves of plates: ill; 16cm (8vo)

98 Farriery improved; or, a complete treatise on the art of farriery: wherein is fully explained the nature and structure of that useful creature, a horse ... / by Henry Bracken ... — A new edition. — London: Printed by H. Harrison, for N. Frobisher ... York, 1790. — 144p, [8] folded leaves of plates: ill; 15cm (18mo)
The various editions of Farriery improved ... published under the name of Henry Bracken by Frobisher were evidently plagiarised and appeared well after Bracken's death in 1764. The "ten elegant cuts, each the full figure of a horse" announced on the titles are present as 10 figures on eight folded plates. The figures are the same as copied from de Saunier for the Lane's and Crosby's plagiarised editions of Taplin improved ... but have been re-drawn differently for the Frobisher editions of Bracken

The gentleman's pocket-farrier
see BURDON, William

99 The traveller's pocket-farrier: or a treatise upon the distempers and common incidents happening to horses upon a journey ... / by Henry Bracken ... — London: Printed for B. Dod ..., 1743. — [8], 151, [9]p; 17cm (12mo)

100 The traveller's pocket-farrier: or a treatise upon the distempers and common incidents happening to horses upon a journey: being very useful for all gentlemen and tradesmen who are obliged to travel the countries / by Henry Bracken ... — The second edition. — London: Printed for B. Dod ..., 1743. — [8], 151, [9]p; 17cm (12mo)

101 The traveller's pocket-farrier: or a treatise upon the distempers and common incidents happening to horses upon a journey: being very useful for all gentlemen and tradesmen who are obliged to travel the countries / by Henry Bracken ... — The third edition, with additions and improvements. — London: Printed for B. Dod ..., 1744. — [8], 150, [10]p; 17cm (12mo)

BRADLEY, Richard, 1688-1732

102 The gentleman and farmer's guide, for the increase and improvement of cattle: viz. lambs, sheep, hogs, ... / by R. Bradley ... — London: Printed by J. Applebee, for W. Mears ..., 1729. — [2], iv, [10], 352p, [4] leaves of plates: ill; 21cm (8vo)

BRADSTREET, John

103 The farmers request: or, a treatise of the particular distempers incident to horses and cows: being a collection of receipts never yet extant / and found out by John Bradstreet ... — Norwich: Printed by William Chase, for the author, 1730. — [2], 53p; 19cm (8vo)
John Bradstreet was a farrier in Suffolk who evidently specialised in treating ailing cows rather than horses. The only other recorded copy of The farmers request ... is that in the BL. Not known to Smith; not in NUC; not in RVC or RCVS. Ex D.J. Spark. See Spark, D.J. (1978) The farmers request by John Bradstreet. Veterinary record, 103, 425-426
Illustration: page 40

BRECKON, H.

104 (A cow doctor). Neu, pob dyn yn feddyg i'w anifail ei hun: y rhan gyntaf ... / gan y cyffeiriwr enwog hwnnw H. Breckon; ac a gyfieithiwyd i'r Cymraeg er lleshad i'r Cymry gan D. T. Jones. — Caernarfon: Argraphwyd gan L.E. Jones, dros yr awdwr, 1820. — 4, 67p; 18cm (12mo)
Illustration: page 41

105 (A sheep doctor). Neu, pob dyn yn feddyg i'w anifail ei hun: y drydedd ran ... / a gyfieithiwyd o'r Saesoneg er lleshad i'r Cymry, gan D.T. Jones. — Caernarfon: Argraphwyd gan L.E. Jones, dros yr awdwr, 1820. — 24p; 18cm (12mo)
A sheep doctor is not credited to Breckon although it is obviously a companion work to A cow doctor from the same translator and publisher. See Ashton, G.M. (1973) Early books in Welsh on veterinary medicine. Veterinary history, 2, 13-23. Not known to Smith
Illustration: page 42

THE
FARMERS REQUEST:
OR, A
TREATISE
OF THE
Particular DISTEMPERS
INCIDENT TO
Horſes and Cows.

Being a COLLECTION of RECEIPTS
Never yet Extant, and found out
BY
JOHN BRADSTREET,
FARRIER of *Wingfield* in *Suffolk.*

NORWICH:
Printed by *Willam Chaſe*, for the AUTHOR.
———
MDCCXXX.

(A COW DOCTOR).

NEU, POB DYN
YN FEDDYG I'W ANIFAIL EI HUN,
Y RHAN GYNTAF,
YN CYNNWYS PEDAIR PENNOD AR DDEG AR HUGAIN
Y rhai sy'n sylwi yn fanol ar ddoluriau,
TUMEWNOL, AC ALLANOL,
GWARTHEG A LLOIAU;
YNGHYD A
MEDDYGINIAETH GYFATEBOL
I BOB CLWYF.
Yr hyn ni eglurwyd erioed i'r Cymry.

YR AIL RAN,
YN CYNNWYS YR UN RHIFEDI O BENNODAU,
Y rhai sy'n sylwi ar ddoluriau, tumewnol ac allanol,
CEFFYLAU, DEFAID, &c.
YNGHYD A
MEDDYGINIAETH GYFERBYNIOL IDDYNT.

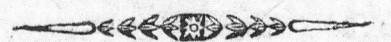

Gan y Cyffeiriwr enwog hwnnw,
H. BRECKON.
Ac a gyfieithiwyd i'r Cymraeg, er lleshâd i'r Cymry.
Gan D. T. Jones.

CAERNARFON:
Argraphwyd gan L. E. Jones, dros yr Awdwr.

1820.

(A SHEEP DOCTOR),

NEU,

POB DYN YN FEDDYG

I'W ANIFAIL EI HUN;

Y DRYDEDD RAN:

YN CYNNWYS,

UN BENNOD AR BYMTHEG,

Y rhai sy'n sylwi yn fanol ar ddoluriau,

TUMEWNOL, AC ALLANOL,

DEFAID AC WYN;

YNGHYD A

MEDDYGINIAETH GYFATEBOL

I BOB CLWYF.

A gyfieithiwyd o'r Saesoneg er lleshâd i'r Cymry,

Gan D. T. Jones.

CAERNARFON:

Argraphwyd gan L. E. Jones, dros yr Awdwr.

1820.

BRETT, Charles C.
106 An anatomical description of the foot of the horse: illustrated by designs ... with a brief treatise on the corns of horses / by Charles C. Brett. — London: Printed for R.H. Laurie, 1829. — 12p, 7 leaves of plates: col.ill; 38cm (4to)
Not known to Smith or to Huth. Not in RVC or RCVS

BRIDGES, Jeremiah
107 No foot, no horse: an essay on the anatomy of the foot of that noble and useful animal a horse ... / by Jeremiah Bridges ... — London: Printed for J. Brindley ... and sold by the author ... and R. Baldwin ..., 1752. — [2], x, 151, [7]p, [2] folded leaves of plates: ill; 20cm (8vo)
Index of remedies, with their prices: p.[4-7]

108 The **BRITISH BIRD FANCIER**: containing instructions for taking, chusing, feeding ... of all the British song & other birds ... — London: T. Hughes, 1824. — 31, [1]p, [1] folded leaf of plates: ill; 18cm (12mo)
Bound with: The new and complete universal vermin-killer. — London: Jones, 1824

BROWN, Sir Edward, 1851-1939
109 British poultry husbandry: its evolution and history / by Sir Edward Brown. — London: Chapman & Hall, 1930. — 350p, [32] leaves of plates: ill, ports.; 23cm

110 Poultry-keeping as an industry for farmers and cottagers / by Edward Brown; illustrated by Ludlow and Sewell. — 3rd ed. — London: Edward Arnold, [1898]. — xii, 128, xvi, [16] leaves of plates: ill; 25cm

111 Races of domestic poultry / by Edward Brown. — London: Edward Arnold, 1906. — xi, 234, xx p: ill; 26cm
Includes 23p of advertisements

BROWN, Robert
112 The compleat farmer: or, the whole art of husbandry ... / by Robert Brown ... — London: Printed for J. Cooke ..., [1759?]-1760. — 117, [5], 120p, [1] leaf of plates: ill; 16cm (12mo)
Pt.2 has separate t.p. and pagination

BROWN, Thomas
113 The complete modern farrier: a manual of veterinary science ... / by Thomas Brown. — London: J.S. Virtue & Co., [1847?]. — [4], 732p, [2], XIV leaves of plates: ill; 22cm (4to)
Additional engraved t.p.

BROWNE, William
114 Browne his fiftie yeares practice ... / by William Browne, gent. — [London]: Printed by Nicholas Okes, & to be sold by Iohn Piper, 1624. — 67 [i.e.63]p: ill; 19cm (4to)
(cont.)

Error in pagination: p.25-28 omitted
Imperfect: prelim. leaves missing. Bound with: The horse-mans honour / [Nicholas Morgan]. — London: I. Marriott, 1620

BUFFON, Georges Louis Leclerc, comte de, 1707-1788
115 [Histoire naturelle. English. Selections] The natural history of the horse: to which is added, that of the ass, bull, cow, ox, sheep, goat and swine ... / translated from the French of the celebrated M. de Buffon. — London: Printed for R. Griffith's ..., 1762. — [2], ii, 340, [2]p, [1] folded leaf of plates: ill; 21cm (8vo)

BULL, B.
116 A compendious system of veterinary instruction: by question and answer ... / by B.Bull. — London: Simpkin, Marshall, and Co., 1835. — [2], vi, 307p; 23cm (4to)

BURDON, William
117 The gentleman's pocket-farrier: shewing how to use your horse on a journey ... / by Capt. William Burdon. — London: Printed for the author by S. Buckley ..., 1730. — [18], 101, [13]p; 17cm (8vo)
Errata: p.[102]

118 The gentleman's pocket-farrier: shewing how to use your horse on a journey ... / by Capt. William Burdon. — London: Printed by E. Owen ..., [173-]. — x, [11]-70, [2]p; 17cm (12mo)
Two copies: one with additional t.p.: The gentleman's pocket-farrier, with large additions and remarks / by Henry Bracken.- 3rd ed.- London: J. Clarke ... S. Birt ... J. Shuckburgh, 1735. The additions and remarks to the pocket farrier / by Henry Bracken are appended with separate t.p. (38, [2]p)

119 The gentleman's pocket-farrier: shewing how to use your horse on a journey ... / by Capt. William Burdon. — London: Printed by John Crage ..., 1732. — x, [11]-74, [2]p; 16cm (12mo)
Ms. notes on binder's blanks

120 The gentleman's pocket-farrier / with large additions and remarks by Dr. Henry Bracken of Lancaster. — The third edition. — London: Printed for J. Clarke ... S. Birt ... and J. Shuckburgh ..., 1735. — [14], 76, [5]p; 16cm (12mo)
By William Burdon. Bracken's remarks occur in footnotes
Two copies: one bound with: The practical farrier / by a Society of Country Gentlemen ... — 3rd ed.- London: E. Owen ... T. Astley ..., 1733

121 The gentleman's pocket-farrier / with large additions and remarks by Dr. Henry Blacken [sic] of Lancaster. — The fourth edition. — London: Printed for, and sold by, J. Clarke ... sold also by S. Birt ... and T. Longman ..., 1737. — [14], 76, [5]p; 18cm (12mo)
By William Burdon

122 The gentleman's pocket-farrier / by Captain Burdon; with large additions and remarks by Dr. Henry Bracken, of Lancaster. — The fourth edition. — London: Printed for W. Johnston ..., 1748. — [14], 76, [5]p; 16cm (12mo)
Bound with: The practical farrier / by a Society of Country Gentlemen ... — 4th ed. — London: T. Longman and T. Astley, 1737

123 The gentleman's pocket-farrier / by Captain Burdon; with large additions and remarks by Dr. Henry Bracken, of Lancaster. — The fifth edition. — London: Printed for W. Johnston ..., 1768. — [14], 76, [5]p; 17cm (12mo)

124 The gentlemans pocket farrier / by Captain Burdon; with large additions and remarks by Dr. Henry Bracken of Lancaster ... — London: Printed for Edwd. Johnston, & sold by Wallis & Stonehouse ..., [177-?]. — [14], 76, [5]p; 17cm (12mo)
Engraved t.p.

BURKE, B. W.
125 A compendium of the anatomy, physiology, and pathology, of the horse: being a clear and familiar description of the various organs and parts ... / by B. W. Burke. — London: Printed for J. Johnson ..., 1806. — vi, [3], viii-xii, 292p, 2 leaves of plates: ill; 18cm (12mo)
Illustration: page 17

BURKE, John French
126 Farming for ladies: or, a guide to the poultry-yard, the dairy and piggery / by the author of "British husbandry". — London: Murray, 1844. — xviii, 511p, [2] leaves of plates: ill; 18cm (12mo)
Added engraved t.p.
Author is J. F. Burke

BURNHAM, George P. (George Pickering), 1814-1902
127 Burnham's new poultry book: a practical treatise on selecting, housing and breeding domestic fowls, and raising poultry and eggs for market / by Geo. P. Burnham. — New York: American News Co.; Boston: N. E. News Co., 1871. — 343p, 16 leaves of plates: ill; 20cm

128 The history of the hen fever: a humorous record / by Geo. P. Burnham. — Boston: J. French; New York: J. C. Derby; Philadelphia: T. B. Peterson, [1855]. — 326p, [1] leaf of plates: ill; 20cm

CAIRD, James, 1816-1892
129 High farming: under liberal covenants, the best substitute for protection / by James Caird. — 5th ed. — Edinburgh: W. Blackwood and Sons, 1849. — ii, 33p, [1] leaf of plates: plan; 22cm (8vo)
Bound with: "Impediments to agricultural improvement" / by Charles R. Colvile. — London: F. & J. Rivington, 1848; A lecture on the science and application of manures / by A. Huxtable. — 5th ed. — London: J. Ridgway, 1847 and Medicines for the cure of the diseases incident to cattle, sheep, etc. / by T. Bellamy. — 9th ed. — Bristol, 1841

CANTELO, William James
130 A practical exposition of the Cantelonian system of hatching eggs, and rearing poultry, game, &c., by hydro-incubation, or top-contact heat ... / by Wm. Jas. Cantelo. — 5th ed., rev. and enl. — London: William Strange, 1851. — 40p; 22cm

CARMAN, Ezra A., 1834-1909
131 Special report on the history and present condition of the sheep industry of the United States / prepared under the direction of D.E. Salmon by Ezra A. Carman, H.A. Heath and John Minto. — Washington: U.S. Department of Agriculture, Bureau of Animal Industry, 1892. — 1000p, 96 leaves of plates: ill; 23cm

132 The **CATTLE PLAGUE.** — [Nottingham: Provincial Horse and Cattle Insurance Co., 1865]. — 4p; 21cm

CAVENDISH, William, Duke of Newcastle
see NEWCASTLE, William Cavendish, Duke of, 1592-1676

133 **CERTAIN ANCIENT TRACTS CONCERNING THE MANAGEMENT OF LANDED PROPERTY REPRINTED.** — London: Printed for C. Bathurst ... and J. Newbery ..., 1767. — [6], 82, viii, 120, viii, v, 6-100p; 21cm (8vo)
Edited by Robert Vansittart. The boke of husbandry and Surveyinge have also been attributed to John Fitzherbert
Contents: Xenophon's Treatise of householde / [translated by G. Hervet] — The boke of husbandry / [attributed to Sir Anthony Fitzherbert] — Surveyinge, 1539 / [attributed to Sir Anthony Fitzherbert]

CHAMBERLIN, W. H.
134 A plan for the employment of labourers / W.H. Chamberlin. — Newport: S. Manning, [18--]. — 7, [1]p; 19cm (4to)
Caption title
Bound with: Every man his own farrier / by Francis Clater. — 20th ed. — London: B. Crosby, 1809

CHOYSELAT, Prudent Le
see PRUDENT LE CHOYSELAT

CLARENDON, Thomas
135 An examination into the true seat and extent of the powers of the horse: with a view to their most advantageous application in draught and burthen ... / by Thomas Clarendon. — Dublin: Hodges and Smith, 1843. — 64p: ill; 23cm (8vo)

CLARK, Bracy, 1771-1860
136 A description of a new horse shoe: which expands to the foot / invented by Bracy Clark. — 2nd ed. — London: Printed for the author, ... and sold by T. & G. Underwood, 1827. — 12p, III leaves of plates: ill; 28cm
Bound with: Stereoplea / by Bracy Clark. — London, 1832

137 A description of two ancient horse-shoes, found near Silbury Hill, in Wiltshire / [by Bracy Clark]. — [London: J. and C. Adlard, printers, 1837]. — 4p, [1] leaf of plates: ill; 28cm
Bound with: Stereoplea / by Bracy Clark. — London, 1832

138 A disclosure of the apparatus for making the new tablet shoe of expansion / [by Bracy Clark]. — 2nd ed. — [London: s.n., 1828?]. — 12p, VI leaves of plates: ill; 28cm
Bound with: Stereoplea / by Bracy Clark. — London, 1832

139 Disorders of the foot of the horse / by Bracy Clark. — London: [s.n.], 1839. — 4p; 28cm
Bound with: Stereoplea / by Bracy Clark. — London, 1832

140 An essay on the canker and corns of horses' feet / by Bracy Clark. — London: Printed for the author, ... and sold by J. Ridgway, 1822. — 18p; 28cm
Bound with: Stereoplea / by Bracy Clark. — L ondon, 1832

141 An essay on the knowledge of the ancients respecting the art of shoeing the horse, and of the probable period of the commencement of this art / by Bracy Clark. — 2nd ed. — London: [s.n.], 1831. — 36p, [1] leaf of plates: ill; 28cm
Caption title
Bound with: Stereoplea / by Bracy Clark. — London, 1832

142 Guide to the shoeing-forge, or plain directions to gentlemen going to have their horses shod ... / by Bracy Clark. — [London: C. Richards, printer, 1830]. — 7p; 28cm
Bound with: Stereoplea / by Bracy Clark. — London, 1832

143 Hippodonomia: or the true structure, laws, and economy, of the horse's foot: also podophthora ... / by Bracy Clark. — 2nd ed., enl. and improved. — London: Printed for the author: sold by T. & G. Underwood, 1829. — 140, [2], 79p, XII [i.e.11] leaves of plates: ill; 28cm (4to)
Bound with 5 other works in vol. with binder's title: Clark's treatises on the horses foot

144 The horse's foot and the horse's shoe / [by Bracy Clark]. — [S.l.: s.n., 185-?]. — [2]p; 26cm
At head of title: From the Empire newspaper
Bound with: Hippodonomia / by Bracy Clark. — London, 1829

145 Index to the sectional figure of the horse: with remarks on certain properties of his general framing / by Bracy Clark. — London: Printed for the author ..., 1813. — 22p, [2] leaves of plates: ill; 28cm
Cover title is: A description of the section of the horse
Without the plate drawn by G. Kirtland. Bound with: Stereoplea / by Bracy Clark. — London, 1832

146 [Letter to Joseph Docwra, and his reply, on the date of the first use of the unilaterally nailed horse shoe] / Bracy Clark. — [London: s.n.], 1836. — [3]p: facsim.; 28cm
Copy 1: Bound with: Hippodonomia / by Bracy Clark. — London, 1829
Copy 2: Bound with: Stereoplea / by Bracy Clark. — London, 1832

147 A new exposition of the horse's hoof / B.C. — [S.l.: s.n.], 1820. — [2]p; 28cm
Notes on dismantling a model hoof
Bound with: Stereoplea / by Bracy Clark. — London, 1832

148 On founder. – Pedicida / [by Bracy Clark]. — [S.l.: s.n., 1834?]. — 4p, [1] leaf of plates: ill; 28cm
The plate is a reproduction of Pl. 3 in Stereoplea
Bound with: Stereoplea / by Bracy Clark. — London, 1832

149 On running frush of horses' feet / [by Bracy Clark]. — 3rd ed. — London: [Richards, printer], 1842. — 8p; 28cm
Bound with: Stereoplea / by Bracy Clark. — London, 1832

150 Remarks on French shoeing [or a review of Jos. Goodwin's A new system of shoeing horses] / by an English shoeing smith [Bracy Clark]. — [S.l.: s.n., 1830?]. — [5]p; 28cm
Bound with: Stereoplea / by Bracy Clark. — London, 1832

151 Remarks with illustrations of the eroded shuttle, or nut-bone, (os nuciforme) of the horse's foot / [by Bracy Clark]. — [London: s.n., 1842?]. — 7p, 1 leaf of plates: ill; 28cm
Bound with: Stereoplea / by Bracy Clark. — London, 1832

152 Review of Wm. Youatt's publication, called 'The horse' / [Bracy Clark]. — [London]: Printed by J.E. Adlard, 1854. — 8p; 28cm
Bound with: Hippodonomia / by Bracy Clark. — London, 1829

153 Ring-bones or ossified cartilages / [by Bracy Clark]. — 2nd ed. — London: [Richards, printer], 1842. — 2p; 28cm
Bound with: Stereoplea / by Bracy Clark. — London, 1832

154 Stereoplea: or, the artificial defence of the horse's foot considered ... / by Bracy Clark. — 2nd ed. — London: Printed for the author; and sold by Renshaw and Rush, 1832. — [2], iv, 52, [1]p, 3 leaves of plates: ill; 28cm (4to)
Bound with 16 other works in vol. with binder's title: Clark's treatises on the horse, 2

155 Testimonies communicated by various persons in favor of the expansion shoe. — London: Printed for the editor, ... and sold by T. & G. Underwood, 1828. — 16p; 28cm
Edited by Bracy Clark
Copy 1: Bound with: Hippodonomia / by Bracy Clark. — London, 1829
Copy 2: Bound with: Stereoplea / by Bracy Clark. — London, 1832

156 The twisted shoe / [by Bracy Clark]. — [S.l.: s.n., 1853?]. — [1]p: ill; 28cm
Bound with: Hippodonomia / by Bracy Clark. — London, 1829

CLARK, Charles

157 An exposure of abuses and malpractices at that institution, called the Royal Veterinary College: stating the injurious effects of its corrupt influence ... / by Charles Clark. — London: J. Ridgway, 1829. — 56p; 21cm (8vo)
Charles Clark was a nephew of Bracy Clark. He came from America and eventually succeeded to his uncle's practice probably in 1828 (Smith, III, 37 & IV, 23). He supports Bracy Clark's criticisms of Coleman and Sewell and of the London College generally, and complains vigorously that the brief, inadequate instruction provided bears no relation to the original plan in 1791 for a three-year course of broadly based training. This copy is bound together with two papers of a similar nature by Clark published in the Farrier and naturalist, nos. 3 and 7, 1828, and three letters published in the Veterinarian in 1839, suggesting that this is likely to have been Clark's own copy. Ex Prof. Cyril Tyler
Illustration: page 50

CLARK, James

158 Observations on the shoeing of horses: together with a new inquiry into the causes of diseases in the feet of horses. In two parts ... / by J. Clark ... — Third edition. — Edinburgh: Printed for William Creech; and sold by T. Cadell, and T. Longman, London, 1782. — x, 11-214p, [1] folded leaf of plates: ill; 22cm (8vo)

159 Observations upon the shoeing of horses: together with a new inquiry into the causes of diseases in the feet of horses. In two parts ... / by J. Clark ... — Edinburgh: Printed for J. Balfour; and T. Cadell, London, 1775. — v, [6]-207p, [1] folded leaf of plates: ill; 21cm (8vo)

160 A treatise on the prevention of diseases incidental to horses: from bad management in regard to stables, food, water, air and exercise. To which are subjoined observations ... / by J. Clark ... — Edinburgh: Printed by W. Smellie for the author; and sold by the booksellers, 1788. — xii, 425, [1]p; 23cm (8vo)
Errata: last p.

161 A treatise on the prevention of diseases incidental to horses: from bad management in regard to stables, food, water, air, and exercise ... / by J. Clark ... — Second edition, corrected and enlarged. — Edinburgh: Printed for the author; and sold by W. Creech [and 3 others], 1790. — xii, 427p; 22cm (8vo)
Binders blanks

EXPOSURE

OF

ABUSES AND MALPRACTICES

At that Institution, called the

Royal
VETERINARY COLLEGE,

STATING

THE INJURIOUS EFFECTS OF ITS CORRUPT INFLUENCE ON THE VETERINARY PROFESSION, AND THE PUBLIC AT LARGE.

WITH A LETTER ADDRESSED TO

THE KING, AS PATRON.

By CHARLES CLARK,

VETERINARY SURGEON.

LONDON:

JAMES RIDGWAY, PICCADILLY.

MDCCCXXIX.

Price One Shilling.

CLATER, Francis, 1756-1823

162 Every man his own cattle doctor; or a practical treatise on the diseases of horned cattle ... / by Francis Clater ... — The fifth edition. — London: Printed for Baldwin, Cradock, and Joy ..., 1817. — xxxii, [33]-384p, [1] leaf of plates: ill; 22cm (8vo)
Copy 1: Provenance: Earl of Kintore (armorial bookplate)
Copy 2: Bound with: Every man his own farrier / by Francis Clater. 23rd ed. — London: W. Lewis for Baldwin, Cradock, and Joy, 1817

163 Every man his own farrier: or, the whole art of farriery laid open ... / by Francis Clater ... — Newark: Printed by J. Tomlinson, for the author, 1783. — xii, 176p; 21cm (8vo)
Ms. notes
Illustration: page 52

164 Every man his own farrier: or, the whole art of farriery laid open ... / by Francis Clater. — The second edition, with corrections and additions. — Newark: Printed by and for J. Tomlinson; and sold by R. Baldwin, and S. Bladon ..., 1786. — xii, 178p; 21cm (8vo)
Some ms. notes

165 Every man his own farrier: or the whole art of farriery laid open ... / by Francis Clater. — The fourth edition, with corrections and additions. — Newark: Printed by and for A. Tomlinson; and sold by R. Baldwin, and S. Bladon ... London, 1791. — xii, 178p; 21cm (8vo)

166 Every man his own farrier: or, the whole art of farriery laid open ... / by Francis Clater. — The sixteenth edition. — Newark: Printed by and for A. Tomlinson; and sold by R. Baldwin ... and B. Crosby and Co. ..., 1806. — XII, 180p; 23cm (8vo)

167 Every man his own farrier; or, the whole art of farriery laid open: containing cures for every disorder a horse is incident to ... / by Francis Clater. — The twentieth edition. — London: Printed, by assignment of A. Tomlinson ... for B. Crosby and Co. ..., 1809. — xi, [1] (blank), 179, [1]p: ill; 18cm (8vo)
Bound with: A plan for the employment of labourers / W.H. Chamberlin. — Newport: S. Manning, [18--]

168 Every man his own farrier: or, the whole art of farriery laid open ... / by Francis Clater ... — The twenty-third edition. — London: Printed by W. Lewis ... for Baldwin, Cradock, and Joy ..., 1817. — XVI, 360p, [1] leaf of plates: port; 22cm (8vo)
Bound with: Every man his own cattle doctor / by Francis Clater. — 5th ed. — London: Baldwin, Cradock, and Joy, 1817

169 Every man his own farrier ... / by Francis Clater. — 31st ed. / edited ... by Edward Mayhew. — London: Longman and Co., 1861. — viii, 362p: ill; 19cm

EVERY MAN
His own FARRIER;

OR,

The whole Art of Farriery laid open:

CONTAINING

CURES for every Disorder that useful Animal, a HORSE, is incident to.

The following are a few of the particular ones:

The POLE-EVIL.	QUITTER BONES.
FISTULAS.	GREASY HEELS.
To take off FALSE QUARTERS and SAND CRACKS.	BONE SPAVINS.
	SCAB, or MANGE.
The FARCY.	The SCAB in Sheep, &c.

TO WHICH IS ADDED,

An APPENDIX:

INCLUDING

Several excellent RECIPES, and the Preparation of many valuable Medicines.

By FRANCIS CLATER,
Late FARRIER, *in* NEWARK.

NEWARK:
Printed by J. TOMLINSON, for the AUTHOR.
M DCC LXXXIII.

[*Entered at Stationers-Hall.*]

170 Clater's Every man his own farrier. — Rev. ... / by D. McTaggart; together with Rarey's Treatment and management of the horse. — London: Milner and Co., [1870?]. — xiv, lxiv, 370p, [2] leaves of plates (1 folded): ill; 13cm
Added, engraved t.p.

CLIFFORD, Christopher

171 The schoole of horsmanship: wherein is discouered vvhat skill and knowledge is required in a good horseman ... / by Christ. Clifford, gent. — Imprinted at London: for Thomas Cadman ..., 1585. — [6], 99 [i.e. 95], [1] (blank) leaves: ill; 18cm (4to)
Provenance: Francis Henry Cripps-Day (armorial bookplate).
Imperfect: leaves 86-87 missing, a few leaves damaged with slight loss of text. The numbering of the leaves is erratic: 1 to 24; 29 to 40; 43(=41); 42 to 49; 54(=50); 51 to 65; 68(=66); 67 to 78; 80(=79); 80 to 99
Illustration: page 54

COLEMAN, Edward, 1765-1839

172 Observations on the formation and uses of the natural frog of the horse: with a description of a patent artificial frog ... / by Edward Coleman ... — [London]: Printed for the author by J. Crowder ... and sold at the Veterinary College ... also, by J. Johnson ..., 1800. — [4], iii, [1] (blank), 23p, [2] folded leaves of plates: ill; 20cm (8vo)

173 Observations on the structure, oeconomy, and diseases of the foot of the horse: and the principles and practice of shoeing / by Edward Coleman ... — London: Printed for the author; and sold at the Veterinary College ... [and others], 1798-1802. — 2v (vii, [1], 128p, [8] leaves of plates; [2], 251, [1] (Errata)p, [30] leaves of plates): ill (some col.); 29cm (4to)
Vol. 1: plates I to IIII each in two states; v.2: plates I to XV each in two states, coloured and outline

COLER, Johann, d.1639

174 M. Iohannis Coleri Oeconomia; oder, Hausbuch ... — Gedruckt zu Wittenberg: bey Wolff Meissner, in vorlegung Paul Helwigs, Buchfuhrers daselbst, 1593-1617. — 5v: ill; 18cm (4to)
Imperfect: pt 4 only. Title and date of publication from NUC pre-1956, v.115, p.60. Rest of the imprint from colophon, this pt. published in 1604. Disbound
Not seen by Smith (I, 217-218)

COLLIER, William

175 Table of doses for the horse & ox; sheep, calf, & pig; dog & cat / by William Collier. — York: William Collier, [18--]. — 1 sheet; 44x29cm

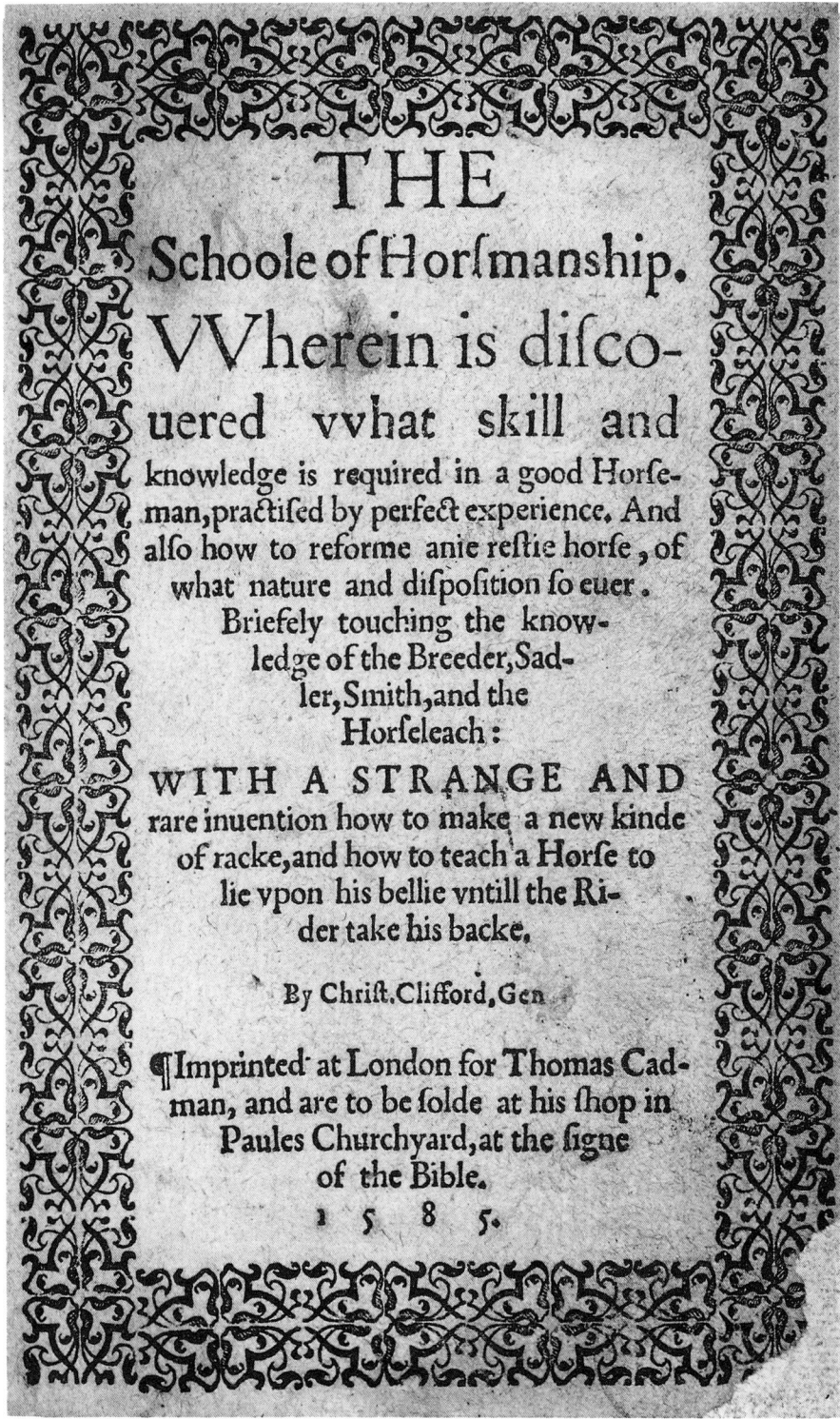

THE
Schoole of Horsmanship.
VVherein is disco-
uered vvhat skill and
knowledge is required in a good Horseman, practised by perfect experience. And
also how to reforme anie restie horse, of
what nature and disposition so euer.
Briefely touching the knowledge of the Breeder, Sadler, Smith, and the
Horseleach:

WITH A STRANGE AND
rare inuention how to make a new kinde
of racke, and how to teach a Horse to
lie vpon his bellie vntill the Rider take his backe.

By Christ. Clifford, Gen.

¶Imprinted at London for Thomas Cadman, and are to be solde at his shop in
Paules Churchyard, at the signe
of the Bible.
1 5 8 5.

COLUMELLA, Lucius Junius Moderatus

176 [De re rustica. English] L. Junius Moderatus Columella of husbandry. In twelve books: and his book concerning trees. Translated into English, with several illustrations from Pliny, Cato, Varro, Palladius, and other antient and modern authors. — London: Printed for A. Millar ..., 1745. — xiv, [14], 600, [8]p; 26cm (4to)
Imperfect: last [8]p Index missing

COLVILE, Charles R.

177 "Impediments to agricultural improvement": considered in a paper read before the Burton-upon-Trent Farmers' Club on Thursday, September 23, 1847 / by Charles R. Colvile. — London: F. & J. Rivington, 1848. — 48p; 22cm (8vo)
Bound with: High farming / by James Caird. — 5th ed. — Edinburgh: W. Blackwood and Sons, 1849

COMBER, T. (Thomas)

178 Real improvements in agriculture: (on the principles of A. Young, esq;) ... / by T. Comber ... — London: Printed for W. Nicoll ..., 1772. — [4], 83p; 22cm (8vo)
Not known to Smith, but see Fussell, II, 94

179 The **COMPLEAT VERMIN-KILLER**: a valuable and useful companion for families ... — London: Printed for Fielding and Walker ..., 1777. — [2], 88p; 21cm (8vo)
Contains an 11-page section on The gentleman farrier; or directions for the purchase, management, & cure of horses

180 The **COMPLETE DOG FANCIER**: or general history of dogs ... — London: T. Hughes, 1824. — 31, [1]p, [1] folded leaf of plates: ill; 18cm (12mo)
Bound with: The new and complete universal vermin-killer. — London: Jones, 1824

181 The **COMPLETE FARMER**; or, general dictionary of agriculture and husbandry: comprehending the most improved methods of cultivation ... — The fifth edition, wholly re-written and enlarged. — London: Printed by Rider and Weed ... for R. Baldwin [and 13 others], 1807. — 2v ([952]p, [59] leaves of plates; [1164]p, [50] leaves of plates): ill; 29cm (4to)
Vol. 1: plates numbered I to LIV, with four plates XIV (part 1, 2, 3 and 4), and 3 out-of-sequence plates of Artificial grasses between plates XLVIII and L; v. 2: plates numbered I to XLIV, with plates 7 and 8 on four leaves, two plates XXIII, two plates XXVI and three plates XXXVIII

182 The **COMPLETE PIGEON AND RABBIT FANCIER**: with instructions for breeding, rearing ... — London: T. Hughes, 1824. — 32p, [1] folded leaf of plates: ill; 18cm (12mo)
Bound with: The new and complete universal vermin-killer. — London: Jones, 1824

183 **CONDY'S DIRECTIONS.** — [London: Condy & Mitchell (Ltd.), 1913?]. — 34, 30xp: ill; 14cm
Title on reverse: Condy's fluid. Veterinary uses. Printed tête-bêche

184 **CONSIDERATIONS ON THE BREED AND MANAGEMENT OF HORSES**: interspersed with some remarks and calculations on the exportation and importation of corn ... — London: Printed for W. Davis ... and J. Wilkie ..., 1778. — [4], vi, 124p; 18cm (8vo)
Errata: p.[i]
C5 is a cancel
This anonymous work not known to Smith or to Huth

CONSTABLE, H. Strickland (Henry Strickland), b.1821
185 The cattle plague: with remarks upon the drainage of farm buildings and stables / by H. Strickland Constable. — 3rd ed. with much additional matter. — York: R. Sunter; London: Hamilton, Adams, & Co, 1866. — 55p; 21cm

COOK, Theodore Andrea, 1867-1928
186 Eclipse & O'Kelly: being a complete history so far as is known of that celebrated English thoroughbred Eclipse (1764-1789) ... / by Theodore Andrea Cook. — London: W. Heinemann, 1907. — xxx, 312, [67] leaves of plates: ill, ports; 26cm
No.95 of a limited ed. of 100

COOK, William, 1849-1904
187 Ducks: and how to make them pay / by William Cook. — St.Mary Cray: W. Cook, [1890]. — vi, 107p, [8] leaves of plates: ill; 19cm

188 Fowls for the times: the history and development of the Orpington fowl / by William Cook. — St.Mary Cray: W. Cook, [1896]. — [20], 165p, [20] leaves of plates: ill, port.; 19cm

189 The horse: its keep & management / by William Cook. — St.Mary Cray: W. Cook, 1891. — viii, 146p: ill; 19cm

190 Pheasants, turkeys and geese: their management for pleasure and profit / by William Cook. — 2nd ed. — London: W. Cook, [189-?]. — [12], 49, [6], 69p, [8] leaves of plates: ill, port; 19cm

191 Practical poultry breeder & feeder: or how to make poultry pay / by William Cook. — London: Published at the Office of the Journal of Horticulture, [1883]. — [iv]-xiii, 108p: ill; 19cm

192 Practical poultry breeder and feeder: or how to make poultry pay / by William Cook. — 9th ed. — London: W. Cook, [1895]. — [16], 234p, [37] leaves of plates: ill, port; 19cm
Preface signed: 1895

COPINEAU, Abbé
193 L'homme rival de la nature: ou l'art de donner l'existence aux oiseaux, & principalement à la volaille par le moyen d'une chaleur artificielle / corrigé d'après l'ouvrage de Réaumur sur cette partie, servant de suite à la Maison rustique. — A Paris: Chez Gay & Gide ..., l'an 3e (1795). — [4], 428p, 4 folded leaves of plates: ill; 20cm (8vo)
By Abbé Copineau

COPLAND, Samuel
194 Agriculture, ancient and modern: a historical account of its principles and practice, exemplified in their rise, progress, and development / by Samuel Copland. — London: Virtue and Co., 1866. — 2v (x, [2], 784p, [26] leaves of plates; iv, 800p, [19] leaves of plates): ill, plans; 29cm
On spine: by the old Norfolk farmer. Samuel Copland wrote under this name in the Mark Lane Express

CORRIGAN, Andrew
195 Theory and practice of modern agriculture: to which is added the breeding, management & diseases of cattle, sheep, pigs, horses and poultry / by Andrew Corrigan. — 2nd ed. — Dublin: "Farmers' gazette", 1858. — viii, 182, 197-216, 183-201, [52], 288-293, xxv-clxxiv p, [7] leaves of plates: ill (some col.); 18cm
Advertisements: p.xxv-clxxiv
Corrigan's work is notable for its engravings of prize animals and breeds of cattle (33), sheep (4), pigs (6), horses (2), and poultry (9), as well as 100 pages of 'profusely illustrated' advertisements

CORTE, Claudio
196 [Il Cavallerizzo. English. Selections] The art of riding: conteining diuerse necessarie instructions ... / written at large in the Italian toong, by Maister Claudio Corte ... Here brieflie reduced into certeine English discourses ... — Imprinted at London: By H. Denham, 1584. — [12], 112p: ill; 18cm (4to)
Translated by Thomas Bedingfield
Reference: STC (2nd ed.) 5797
Imperfect: p.9-16 & p.87-88 missing. Disbound
Illustration: page 58

COUNTRY GENTLEMAN
197 The complete grazier: or, Gentleman and farmer's directory: containing the best instructions for buying, breeding and feeding cattle ... / written by a country gentleman, and originally designed for private use. — London: Printed for J. Almon ..., 1767. — xii, 252p; 18cm (12mo)
Not known to Smith or to Fussell. Not in RVC or RCVS

198 A new system of agriculture: or, a plain, easy, and demonstrative method of speedily growing rich ... / by a country gentleman. — The second edition. — London: Printed for A. Millar ..., 1755. — 240p; 17cm (12mo)

THE
Art of Riding, conteining diuerse necessarie instructions, demonstrations, helps, and corrections apperteining to horssemanship, not heretofore expressed by anie other Author:

Written at large in the Italian toong, by Maister Claudio Corte, a man most excellent in this Art.

Here brieflie reduced into certeine English discourses to the benefit of Gentlemen and others desirous of such knowledge.

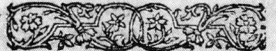

Imprinted at London by H. Denham.
1584.

The **COUNTRY GENTLEMAN'S COMPANION**
see MARKHAM, Gervase, 1568?-1637

199 The **COW DOCTOR**: a practical treatise on the diseases of horned cattle and sheep ... — London: Richardson and Son, 1844. — 323, [1]p: ill; 13cm (8vo)
Additional, engraved t.p.: The modern pocket cattle doctor. — Derby: Thomas Richardson & Son, 1844

COX, Nicholas
200 The gentleman's recreation: in four parts ... whereto is added, a perfect abstract of all the forest-laws ... — The sixth edition with large additions. — London: Printed for N.C. and sold by J. Wilcox ... [and 3 others], 1721. — [4], iv, 438, [2], 115, [9]p, [5] leaves of plates (4 folded): ill; 21cm (8vo)
Dedication signed by Nicholas Cox
Several errors in pagination

CRAMP, William
201 Hints to dairy farmers: being an account of the food, and extraordinary produce of a cow ... / by William Cramp ... — The second edition, with two additional years. — London: Printed and sold by B. McMillan ... sold also by Sherwood, Neely & Jones ... and Baxter, Lewes, 1813. — 44p; 22cm (8vo)

CRAWSHEY, John
202 The good husband's jewel: containing plain and easy directions how to know the means whereby horses, beasts, &c. come to have many diseases ... — [S.l.: s.n., 17--?]. — 32p; 18cm (4to)
By John Crawshey
Illustration: page 60

CRIPPS-DAY, Francis Henry
203 The manor farm / by Francis Henry Cripps-Day. To which are added reprint-facsimiles of The boke of husbandry: an English translation ... by Walter of Henley ascribed to Robert Grosseteste ... and The booke of thrift: containing ... Hosebonderie by James Bellot ... — London: B. Quaritch Ltd., 1931. — xxxviii, 114, [66]p, [1] leaf of plates: facsims; 22cm

CROAD, A. C.
204 The Langshan fowl: its history and characteristics with some comments on its early opponents / [by A.C. Croad]. — 3rd ed. — London: Bowers Brothers, 1889. — [2], 122p, [6] leaves of plates: ill, map; 21cm

CULLEY, George, 1735-1813
205 Observations on live stock: containing hints for choosing and improving the best breeds of the most useful kinds of domestic animals / by George Culley, farmer at Fenton, Northumberland. — London: Printed for G.G.J. & J. Robinson ..., 1786. — [8], 195, [2]p; 22cm (8vo)
The first edition not seen by Smith. This copy ex-Fussell who (II, 128) gives the date as 1787

The Good Husband's JEWEL.

Containing, Plain and Easy *Directions* how to know the Means whereby Horses, Beasts, &c. come to have many Diseases; the Way to cure them perfectly, and with little Cost or Charge.

Written by a very Skilful *Hand*, who had his Knowledge, not by reading or perusing any Book, but by above Thirty Years Experience, besides the Practice of his Ancestors; being very useful for all Country Men, whereby they may be able to save their *Cattle*.

With an Admirable and Safe Way for Gelding and Spaving both Male and Female, approved by the Testimony of divers Worthy Gentlemen, both Knights and Esquires, in the Counties of *York, Lincoln,* &c.

Also Proper *Directions,* for the Destroying all Manner of VERMIN in HOUSES, GARDENS, FIELDS, &c.

To which is added,

The true Tutor for Pacing of HORSES.

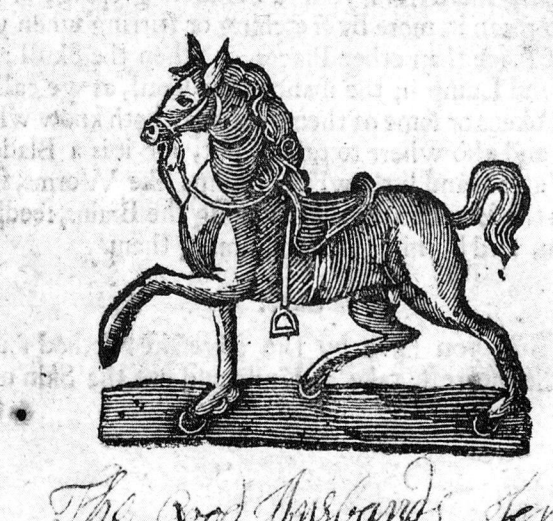

The good Husbands Jewel

206 Observations on live stock: containing hints for choosing and improving the best breeds of the most useful kinds of domestic animals / by George Culley, farmer, Northumberland. — The second edition, altered and enlarged. — London: Printed for G.G. & J. Robinson ..., 1794. — vii, [1], xx, [21]-222p, [3] leaves of plates (1 folded): ill; 22cm (8vo)

207 Observations on live stock: containing hints for choosing and improving the best breeds of the most useful kinds of domestic animals / by George Culley, farmer, Northumberland. — The third edition, altered and enlarged. — London: Printed for G.G. & J. Robinson ..., 1801. — vii, [1] (blank), xx, [21]-222p, [3] leaves of plates (1 folded): ill; 21cm (8vo)

CUNDALL, J.
208 The new cow doctor: containing many valuable receipts ... / by J. Cundall, late of Brandsby. — [S.l.: s.n., 1804]. — 16p; 16cm (8vo)
This small tract by Cundall – price one penny – is undated but the paper is watermarked 1804. Not known to Smith or to Fussell

DACRE, B. (Bartholomew)
209 Testimonies in favor of salt as a manure: and a condiment for horse, cow, and sheep ... / by the Rev. B. Dacre. — Manchester: Printed for the author ... sold by Longman, Hurst, and Co. [and 6 others], 1825. — 288, [2]p; 22cm (8vo)

DALE, John Stamper
210 Veterinary receipt book: for the use of farmers, horse proprietors ... / by John Stamper Dale. — Kirby Moorside: [s.n., 1869]. — 84p; 18cm
John Stamper Dale is described as 'Late veterinary surgeon to the Rosedale and Ferryhill Iron Stone Company'. The Preface is dated 1869

DARBY, Joseph
211 Sheep: their varieties, points and characteristics: with how to breed and graze for profit ... / by Joseph Darby. — London: Dean and Son, [1878?]. — [6], 106p, [6] leaves of plates: ill; 18cm

212 **DARLUNIAD O GLWYF DINYSTRIOL Y'MHLITH LLOI BYCHAIN ...** — Llanerchymedd: E. Jones, 1824. — 1 sheet; 21x16cm

DAUBENTON, Louis Jean Marie, 1716-1799
213 Instruction pour les bergers: et pour les propriétaires de troupeaux ... / par Daubenton; publiée ... par J.B. Huzard ... — Quatrième édition, augmentée. — A Paris: De l'imprimerie et dans la librairie de Madame Huzard ..., 1810. — lxxx, 430p, XXII leaves of plates: ill; 21cm (8vo)

DAY, SON AND HEWITT
214 Price list / Day, Son & Hewitt. — London: Day, Son & Hewitt, [19--]. — 59p: ill; 17cm

DE GRAY, Thomas

215 The compleat horseman and expert ferrier: in two bookes ... / by Thomas de Gray esquire. — London: Printed by Thomas Harper, and are to be sold by Nicholas Fussell ..., 1639. — [30], 356, [5]p, [1] leaf of plates: ill; 27cm (4to)
Reference: STC (2nd ed.) 12206a

216 The compleat horse-man, and expert ferrier: in two bookes ... / by Thomas de Grey [sic], esquire. — The second edition corrected, with some additions. — London: Printed for Thomas Harper and Nicholas Fussell, 1651. — [30], 631, [13]p, [1] leaf of plates: ill; 18cm (4to)

217 **DELLA DOMATIONE DEL POLEDRO**: del suo amaistramento ... / da incerto philosopho antichamente scritta ... novamente percio venuta nelle mani del Biondo, da lui tradutta in lingua materna per uostra consolatione, & data in luce. — In Vinegia: Appresso il Biondo, 1549. — 21, [2] leaves; 15cm (8vo)
Provenance: J. Gomez de la Cortina (armorial bookplate)
Bound with: Opera de l'arte del malscalcio / di Lorenzo Rusio. — In Venetia: Per Michele Tramezino, 1548
Imperfect: leaves 17-20 missing

DE SAUNIER, Jean
see SAUNIER, Jean de

DE SOLLEYSEL, Jacques
see SOLLEYSEL, Jacques de, 1617-1680

DICK, William, 1793-1866
218 Occasional papers on veterinary subjects / by William Dick; with a memoir by R.O. Pringle. — Edinburgh; London: W. Blackwood and Sons, 1869. — 12, cxi, [1] (blank), 501p: port; 23cm

DICKSON, Adam, 1721-1776
219 The husbandry of the ancients / by Adam Dickson ... — Edinburgh: Printed for J. Dickson, and W. Creech ... and G. Robinson, and T. Cadel, London, 1788. — 2v (xxiii, 527; vi, 494p); 22cm (8vo)

DICKSON, R. W.
220 An improved system of management of live stock and cattle: or a practical guide to the perfecting and improvement of the several breeds and varieties of agricultural stock, and domestic animals ... / by R.W. Dickson. — London: Printed for Thomas Kelly, [1822-1824]. — 2v (iv, 504p, [15] leaves of plates; [2], 510p, [19] leaves of plates): col.ill, port; 27cm (fol.)
Additional engraved t.p. with title: Improved live stock and cattle management
Published in parts
All plates are hand-coloured except the engraved portrait frontispiece and additional t.p. in v. 1. The plate listed to face p. 120 of v. 1 was not issued, the engraving of Internal viscera of cow having been included on the plate facing p.97

221 Practical agriculture; or, a complete system of modern husbandry: with the methods of planting, and the management of live stock / by R.W. Dickson ... — London: Printed for Richard Phillips ... by R. Taylor and Co. ..., 1805. — 2v: ill (some col.); 28cm (4to)
Vol. 1: [2], xix, [21], 618, [1]p, LIII leaves of plates (two folded); v. 2: [11], 584-1265, [1]p, XXXIV leaves of plates
Each plate faces an explanatory text, printed on leaves which are not included in the pagination (except plates I and XXXVIII in v. 1). Vol. 2 plates V to XX (of grasses) and plates I and XXIV to XXXIII (of breeds of cattle, sheep, horses and pigs) are hand-coloured

DICKSON, Walter B.
222 Poultry, their breeding, rearing, diseases and general management / by Walter B. Dickson; with corrections and large additions by Mrs. Loudon. — New ed.; incorporating the treatise of Bonington Moubray. — London: Bohn, 1853. — xii, 263p, [11] leaves of plates: ill (one col.); 19cm
Bonington Moubray is the pseud. of John Lawrence

DIDEROT, Denis, 1713-1784
223 [Maréchal ferrant and maréchal grossier]. — [A Paris: Chez Briasson ... Le Breton ..., 1769]. — [4]p, VII, X leaves of plates (some folded): ill; 42cm (fol.)
Extract from v.7 of the Encyclopédie
Illustration: page 64

DIGBY, Henry
224 How to make £50 a year by keeping ducks; also the breeding and management of the most useful varieties of geese and turkeys / by Henry Digby. — 2nd ed. — Huddersfield: H. Digby, [1893?]. — 177, [1]p, [2] leaves of plates: ill, port.; 19cm

DIXON, Edmund Saul, 1809-1893
225 Ornamental and domestic poultry: their history and management / by Edmund Saul Dixon. — 2nd ed. rev. and enl. — London: "Gardeners' Chronicle", 1850. — xxxii, 404p: ill; 18cm (8vo)
Repr. from the Gardeners' chronicle and agricultural gazette with additions

226 The **DOMESTIC POULTRY INSTRUCTOR**: being a complete guide ... to which is added, instructions in the management of bees ... — London: T. Hughes, [1824?]. — 32p, [1] folded leaf of plates: ill; 18cm (12mo)
Bound with: The new and complete universal vermin-killer. — London: Jones, 1824

DONALDSON, John, 1799-1876
227 British agriculture: containing the cultivation of land, management of crops, and the economy of animals / by J. Donaldson. — London: Atchley & Co., 1860. — vi, [2], 835p, [1] leaf of plates: ill; 28cm
G.E. Fussell's copy (signature). In 3 v.

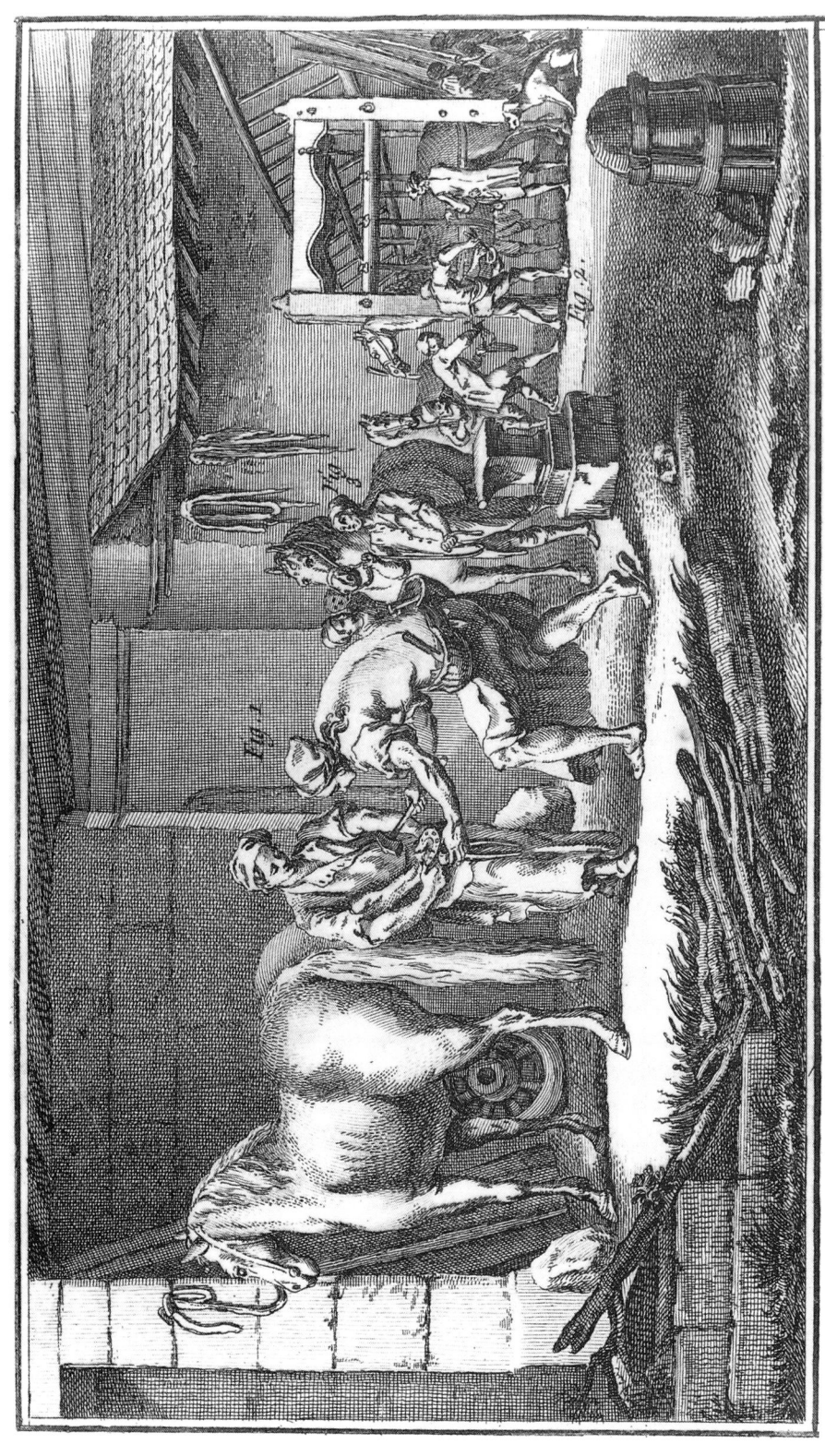

DOUGLAS, William
228 Horse-shoeing as it is and as it should be / by William Douglas. — London: J. Murray, 1873. — xii, [2], 161p, [2] leaves of plates: ill (some col.); 20cm

DOWNING, J. (Joseph)
229 A treatise on the disorders incident to horned cattle: comprising a description of their symptoms ... to which are added receipts ... / by J. Downing. — Printed and sold at Stourbridge: Sold also by T. Hurst, Messrs. Longman and Rees ... and Messrs. Rivington ... London, 1797. — xii, 131, [3], xiii, [2]p; 22cm (8vo)
Errata: p.[3]
A list of subscribers: p.[i]-xiii, [1]
Statement of responsibility transposed
Ms notes laid in; binders blanks

230 A treatise on the disorders incident to horned cattle: comprising a description of their symptoms ... to which are added, receipts ... / by J. Downing. — Kidderminster: Printed and sold by G. Gower: sold also by Messrs. Longman, Hurst, Rees, and Orme, London, [1807?]. — 12, [2], [17]-145p; 24cm (8vo)
Statement of responsibility transposed

231 A treatise on the disorders incident to horned cattle: comprising a description of their symptoms ... to which are added, receipts ... — Newtown: [s.n.], 1836. — [2], iv, [2], 152p, [4] leaves of plates: ill; 17cm (8vo)
By J. Downing
The text of Downing's Treatise is largely derived from the work by Topham (631). The late (1836) edition appears to have been pirated and is not credited to either author. Some new material has been added, together with four plates: A Tees-water Bull, belonging to George Coates ... 1793 (bound as a frontispiece); A Tees-water Heifer ...; A Ram of the Heath Breed; and Staffordshire Boar. This late edition not known to Smith. See also Rowlands (537)

DOYLE, Martin
232 The illustrated book of domestic poultry / edited by Martin Doyle. — London: Routledge, 1854. — iv, 251, 113, [3]p, [20] leaves of plates: col.ill; 23cm
Martin Doyle is the pseud. of William Hickey
Originally published in fascicles under various titles
Imperfect: lacking one plate

233 The illustrated book of domestic poultry / edited by Martin Doyle. — New ed. — London: G. Routledge & Sons, [1870]. — [iii]-vi, 251, 113, [1], 14p, [16] leaves of plates: col.ill; 20cm
Martin Doyle is the pseud. of William Hickey

DRINKWATER, Samuel
234 Every man his own farrier: wherein are set down, in a clear and intelligible manner, the accidents and diseases to which horses are liable, and the method of cure / by Samuel Drinkwater. — Hereford: Printed by W.H. Parker ..., 1796. — [2], ii, [2], 185p; 22cm (8vo)

DRURY, Charles
235 Recent and important national discoveries, of a new system of farming, feeding of cattle: manuring of land, &c. at half the usual expense ... / by Charles Drury ... — The third edition, greatly enlarged. — London: Published for the author, by Baldwin, Cradock and Joy ..., 1815. — 200p; 22cm (8vo)

E.R.
236 The experienced farrier, or, Farring compleated: in two books physical and chyrurgical. Being pleasure to the gentleman, and profit to the countrey-man ... / by E.R. Gent. — London: Printed for Rich. Northcott ..., 1678. — [4], 161, [21], 54, 159, [39]p, [1] folded leaf of plates: ill; 20cm (4to)
Errata: p.[18] (3rd group) and p.[38] at the end
Second pt. has separate t.p.
Illustration: page 67

237 The experienced farrier, or, farring compleated: in two books physical and chyrurgical. Bringing pleasure to the gentleman, and profit to the countrey-man ... / by E.R. Gent. — The second edition much enlarged and amended ... — London: Printed by Richard Northcott ..., 1681. — [16], 418, [40]p, [1] leaf of plates: ill; 22cm (4to)
Second pt. has separate t.p. dated 1680, "The second impression much enlarged and amended by A.O."
Errata: on p.[16] (1st group) and on p.[39]
T.p. repaired with some loss of text

238 The experienc'd farrier: or, a compleat treatise of horsemanship: in two books; physical and chyrurgical. Fitted to the use, not only of gentlemen, but of all farriers ... / by E.R. Gent. — The second edition much enlarged ... — London: Printed for W. Whitwood ... and A. Feltham ..., 1691/2. — [16], 418, [40]p; 22cm (4to)
Second pt. has separate t.p. dated 1680, "The second impression much enlarged and amended by A.O."
Errata on p.[16] (1st group) and on p.[39]
Reference: Wing R14
Imperfect: frontispiece missing
Smith (I, 332) had only seen the 'Fourth Edition' of The experienced farrier ... (1720) and was not aware of any editions before 1682

EARL, Abel
239 A treatise on the disorders of neat cattle: with the causes, symptoms, and mode of cure / by Abel Earl. — Carlisle: Printed for the author, 1835. — [2], xxiii, [24]-185, [1], 2p; 18cm (12mo)

EDWARDS, Kinard B. (Kinard Baghot), b.1848
240 Poultry keeping on a large or small scale: showing how the French produce fowls and eggs by the thousand at a cost of one penny per dozen: fowls 3d. per pound. Part 1. / by Kinard B. Edwards. — [Hinckley]: K.B. Edwards, [1878]. — 23p; 18cm

THE EXPERIENCED FARRIER, OR, Farring Compleated.

IN TWO BOOKS
PHYSICAL and CHYRURGICAL
BEING
Pleasure to the Gentleman, and Profit to the Countrey-man.

IN WHICH

You have the Whole Body, Sum and Substance of it, in one Entire Volume, in so Full and Ample Manner, that there is Little or Nothing more Material to be Added thereto.

For here is Contained

Everything that belongs to a True HORSE-MAN, GROOM, FARRIER, or HORSE-LEACH, *Viz.* BREEDING; The Manner How, The Sea on When, The Place Where, The Colours, Marks and Shapes of all Stallions and Mares, and what are Fit for Generation; The Feeder, Rider, Keeper, Ambler and Buyer; As also the making of several Precious Drinks, Suppositories, Pills, Purgations, Scourings, Ointments, Salves, Powders, Waters, Charges, Balls, Perfumes, And Directions how to use them for all Inward and Outward Diseases.

ALSO

The PARING and SHOOING of all manner of HOOFES, and in what Point that ART doth Consist. The Prices and Vertues of most of the Principal Drugs, both Simple and Compound belonging to *Farring*, (and where you may buy them) *Viz. Roots, Barks, Woods, Flowers, Fruits, Seeds, Juices, Gums, Rozins, &c.* As also a large Table of the Vertues of most Simples set down Alphabetically; And many Hundreds of Words Placed one after another, for the Cure of all Diseases; With many New Receipts of Excellent Use and Value, never yet Printed before in any Author.

By E. R. Gent.

LONDON, Printed for *Rich. Northcott* Adjoyning to St. *Peters* Alley in *Cornhill*, and at the *Mariner and Anchor* upon *New-Fish-street Hill*, near *London*-bridge. 1678.

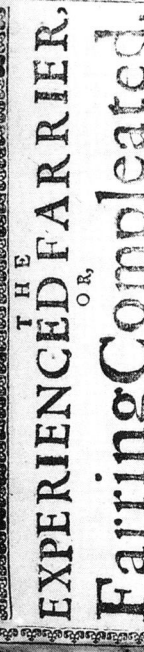

E.R. 1678 (236)

241 **EGGS ALL THE YEAR ROUND AT FOURPENCE PER DOZEN, AND CHICKENS AT FOURPENCE PER POUND**. — 2nd ed. — Glasgow: J. Maclehose; London: Macmillan, 1876. — 95p; 18cm

242 **EGGS ALL THE YEAR ROUND AT FOURPENCE PER DOZEN, AND CHICKENS AT FOURPENCE PER POUND**. — 3rd ed. — Glasgow: J. Maclehose, 1878. — 95p; 17cm

ELLIS, William, d.1758

243 A compleat system of experienced improvements: made on sheep, grass-lambs, and house-lambs ... / by William Ellis, of Little Gaddesden, in Hertfordshire. — London: Printed for T. Astley; and sold by R. Baldwin ... and E. Nicolson ..., 1749. — viii, [24], 384p; 21cm (8vo)

244 Every farmer his own farrier: or the best methods of preventing and curing the injuries and diseases ... / by William Ellis, late a farmer at Little Gaddesden ... — London: Printed for L. Davis and C. Reymers ..., 1759. — vi, [14], 139p; 18cm (8vo)
Horizontal chain lines
A2 and A3 misbound behind a2
Illustration: page 69

ELLSWORTH, Henry W., 1814-1864

245 The American swine breeder: a practical treatise on the selection, rearing and fattening of swine / by Henry W. Ellsworth. — Boston: Week, Jordan and Co., 1840. — 304p, [2] leaves of plates: ill; 17cm (8vo). — (Farmers' series; vol.1)

ESTIENNE, Charles, 1504-1564

246 Maison rustique, or, The countrey farme. / Compyled in the French tongue by Charles Stevens, and Iohn Liebault ... And translated into English by Richard Surflet ... — Now newly reuiewed, corrected, and augmented ... / by Gervase Markham. — London: Printed by Adam Islip for John Bill, 1616. — [18], 732, [22]p: ill; 29cm (fol.)
Reference: STC (2nd ed.) 10549
Illustration: page 70

EVANS, Ernest

247 The biology of poultry keeping or the domestic fowl: its history, anatomy, food, reproduction and breeding / by Ernest Evans. — Brierfield: A.R. Kenyon; Burnley: Utility Poultry Society, 1899. — xiv, [2], 108p: ill; 22cm

248 The **EXPRESS: OR, EVERY MAN HIS OWN DOCTOR** ... / by J. Arundel & Sons. — 10th ed. enl. — Gainsborough: J. Arundel & Sons, 1827. — iv, [5]-48p; 18cm (12mo)

EVERY FARMER HIS OWN FARRIER:

OR

The best Methods of preventing and curing the Injuries and Diseases of that truly serviceable Creature a HORSE:

Laid down in

A different Manner from what has hitherto appeared on this Subject:

Chiefly from

CASES and FACTS;

And performed by the cheapest Ingredients.

By WILLIAM ELLIS,
Late a Farmer at *Little Gaddesden*, near *Hempstead*, in *Hertfordshire*:
Author of the *Modern Husbandman*, and other Works.

LONDON:
Printed for L. DAVIS and C. REYMERS, against *Gray's-Inn, Holborn.* 1759.

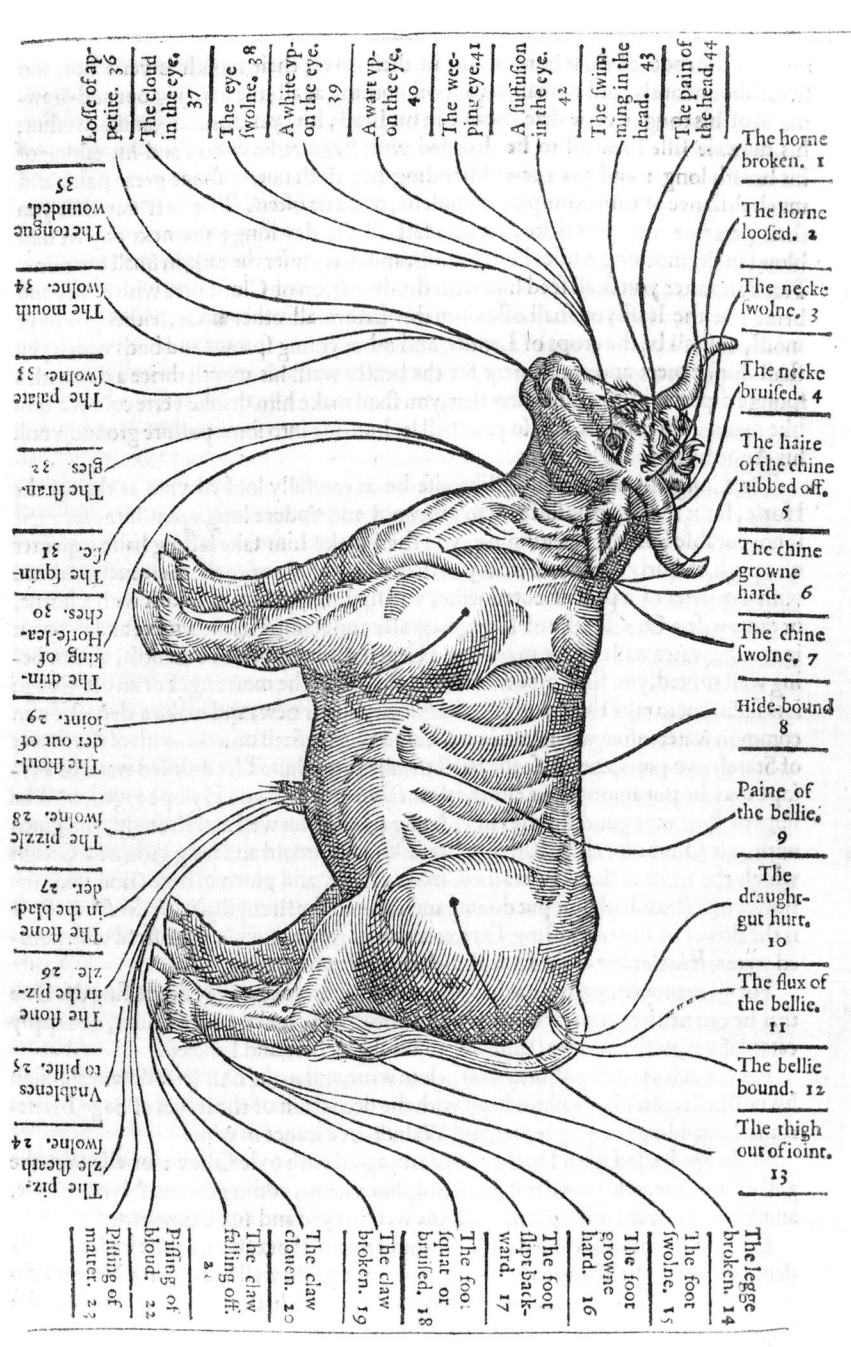

F.M.
249 The jockey's guide: and farrier's companion: containing the best directions for breeding, buying, and preservation of horses ... / by F.M. Gent. — London: Printed for Henry Rhodes ..., 1687. — [11], 216p: ill; 15cm (12mo)
Reference: Smith, I, 344-345
Imperfect: p.195-214 missing

FAIRBAIRN, John
250 A treatise upon breeding, rearing and feeding Cheviot and Black-faced sheep in high districts: with some account of – and a complete cure for, that fatal malady the rot ... / by a Lammermuir farmer. — Berwick-upon-Tweed: Printed for the author, 1823. — xli, [3], 196p; 22cm (4to)
By John Fairbairn

FAIRFAX, Thomas
251 The complete sportsman; or, Country gentleman's recreation: containing the whole arts of breeding and managing game cocks ... / by Thomas Fairfax, esq. — London: Printed for J. Cooke ..., [1760?]. — vi, [7]-240p, [1] leaf of plates: ill; 18cm (12mo)
24p. advertisements for J. Cooke bound in

252 The new complete sportsman; or, the town and country gentleman's recreation: containing, among the various diversions ... angling in all its various branches, the breeding and managing game cocks ... / the whole revised, corrected and improved, by George Morgan, esq. assisted by many experienced gentlemen ... — London: Printed for Alex. Hogg ..., [1785?]. — iv, 302 [i.e.202], [2]p, [1] leaf of plates: ill; 17cm (12mo)
A revision of Thomas Fairfax's The complete sportsman
Error in pagination: p.202 misnumbered as 302

253 **FARRALL'S PATENT VESICANT.** — Dublin: J.J. Farrall, [1869?]. — 12p; 19cm

254 The **FARRIER AND NATURALIST.** — London: Published for the editor, by Simpkin and Marshall, 1828-1830. — 21cm (8vo)
Vol.2 is entitled: The Farrier and naturalist; or, horseman's chronicle; and v.3 is: The Hippiatrist, and veterinary journal
Holdings: Vol.1, no.1 (Jan.1828) — v.3, no.60 (Dec.15, 1830)

FERGUSON, George
255 Ferguson's illustrated series of rare and prize poultry, including comprehensive essays upon all classes of domestic fowl / by G. Ferguson; drawn and colored ... by C.J. Culliford. — London: G. Ferguson ... C.J. Culliford ..., 1854. — x, 372, 5, [1]p, [18] leaves of plates: ill.(some col.); 22cm

FERON, John

256 A complete treatise on farriery: comprising the transactions, or, modern practice of the veterinary art ... / by J. Feron ... — London: Printed for J.J. Stockdale ..., 1810. — [2], 15, [1], 496p, [1] leaf of plates: ill; 24cm (8vo)

257 A new system of farriery: including a systematic arrangement of the external structure of the horse ... / by John Feron. — London: Printed by Betham & Warde ... for J. Johnson ..., 1803. — xv, [1], 272, [1]p, [11] leaves of plates: ill; 29cm (4to)
Errata: p.[1] (2nd group)

FERRARO, Giovanni Battista, d.1569?

258 Delle razze: disciplina del cavalcare ... / per il S. Giouambattista Ferraro cauallerizzo napoletano. — In Napoli: Appresso Mattio Cancer, 1560. — [4], 123, [1] leaves; 21cm (4to)

FIASCHI, Cesare, 1523-ca.1590

259 Trattato del modo dell'imbrigliare, maneggiare, & ferrare cavalli: diuiso in tre parti ... / di M. Cesare Fiaschi gentil'huomo ferrarese. — In Vineggia: Per Francesco de Leno, 1563. — 103, [5] leaves: ill; 15cm (8vo)
Date of imprint from colophon
The illustrations include 40 whole-page woodcuts of horse bits

FIELD, John, d.1839

260 Posthumous extracts from the veterinary records of the late John Field / edited by his brother William Field. — London: Longman, Brown, Green and Longmans, 1843. — x, 236p; 23cm (4to)

FITZHERBERT, John, 1460-ca.1531

261 The boke of husbandry. — Imprynted at London: ... Thomas Berthelet ..., 1534. — [6], 90 leaves; 14cm (8vo)
By: John or Sir Anthony Fitzherbert
Imprint from colophon
Reference: STC (2nd ed.) 10996
Illustration: page 73

262 [The boke of husbandry] The book of husbandry / by Master Fitzherbert. — Repr. from the ed. of 1534 / and edited with an introduction, notes, and glossarial index by the Rev. Walter W. Skeat. — London: Published for the English Dialect Society by Trubner & Co., 1882. — xxx, [1], 167p; 23cm. — (English Dialect Society. series D: miscellaneous)
By: John or Sir Anthony Fitzherbert

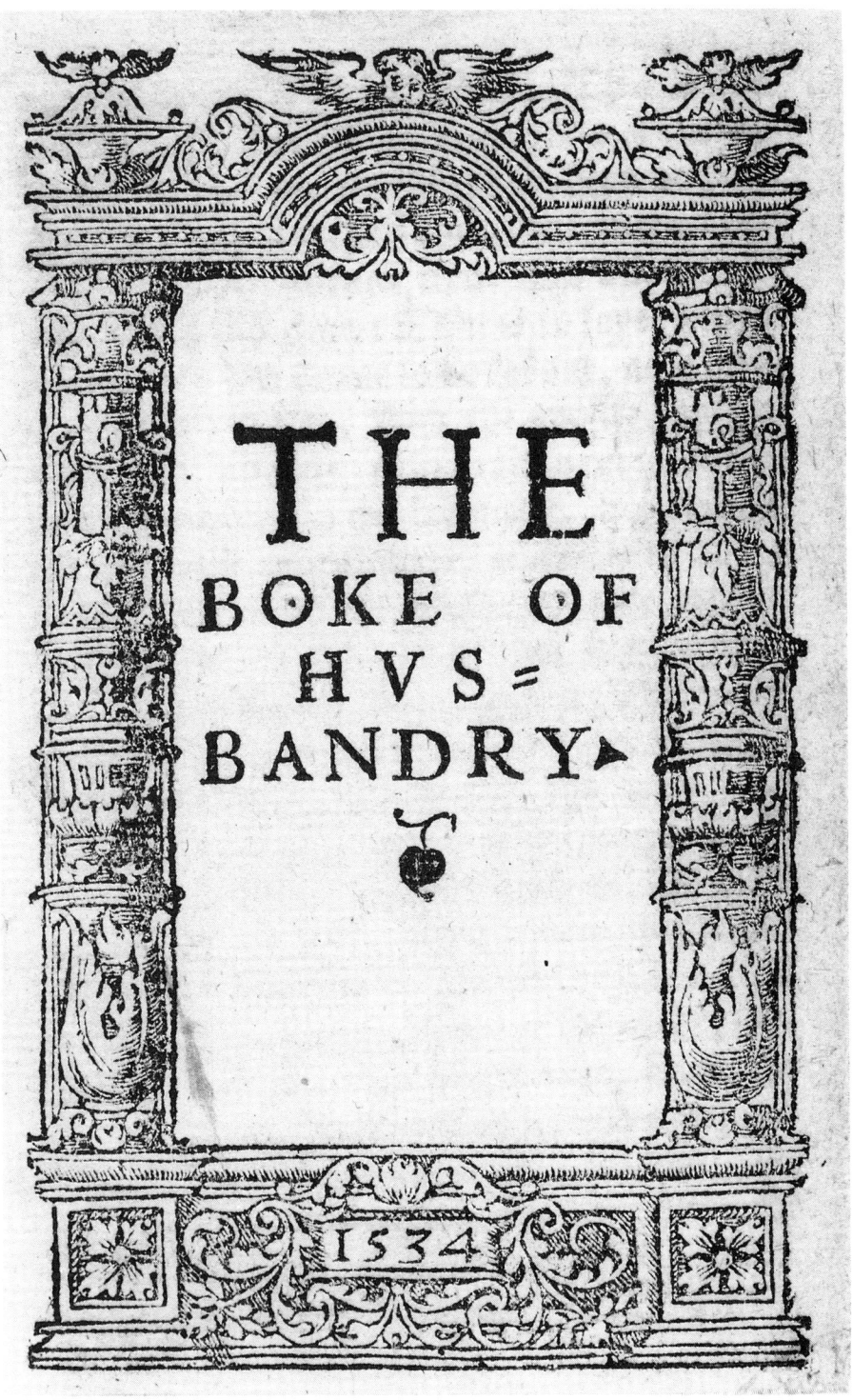

263 [The boke of husbandry] Fitzharberts booke of husbandrie: devided into foure seuerall bookes ... — And now newlie corrected, amended, and reduced, into a more pleasing forme of English then before. — At London: Printed by I.R. for Edward White ..., 1598. — [6], 199, [9]p: ill; 18cm (4to)
Dedication signed: I.R. (James Roberts ?). By: John or Sir Anthony Fitzherbert
Imperfect: p.121-122 (R 1) missing

FLEMING, George, 1833-1901
264 Animal plagues: their history, nature, and prevention / by George Fleming. — London: Baillière, Tindall & Cox, 1871-1882. — 2v ([2], xxxiv, 548, 32; xii, 539p); 23cm
Imprint under label in v. 1: Chapman and Hall
Vol. 1. From B.C. 1490 to A.D. 1800 — v. 2. From A.D. 1800-1844

265 A text-book of veterinary obstetrics: including the diseases and accidents incidental to pregnancy ... / by George Fleming. — London: Baillière, Tindall & Cox, 1878. — xxix, 759p: ill; 24cm

FLINT, Charles L., 1824-1889
266 Milch cows and dairy farming: comprising the breeds, breeding, and management ... / by Charles L. Flint. — A new ed. — Boston: Crosby, Nichols, Lee & Co., 1860. — 426p: ill; 21cm

FLINT, William
267 A treatise on the breeding, training, and management of horses: with practical remarks & observations on farriery ... / by Wm. Flint ... — Hull: Printed for the author, by Topping and Dawson ... sold by Longman, Hurst, Rees, Orme and Brown [and 3 others], London, 1815. — xx, [21]-144p; 20cm (12mo)
Errata inserted
Author's signature on t.p.

FORESTER, Brooke
268 The pocket farrier, or approved receipts: collected from different authors ... — Shrewsbury: Printed by W. Williams, [1770?]. — 34p; 12cm (12mo)
By Brooke Forester
Interleaved with ms. notes
Illustration: page 75

269 **FORTUNES FROM EGGS**: being a collection of actual results obtained by the leading poultry breeders and the most wide-awake poultry keepers / done into a book by the Karswood Company. — Manchester: The Company, 1919. — 128p: ill (some col.); 19cm

FOSSE, Etienne Guillaume La
see LA FOSSE, Etienne Guillaume, d.1765

THE
POCKET-FARRIER,

OR

APPROVED RECEIPTS

COLLECTED

From Different Authors;
With an Intent to Cure or Aſſiſt, any immediate Accidents that may happen to a HORSE, till further help can be got.

A ſtich in time, ſaves nine.

Old Prov·

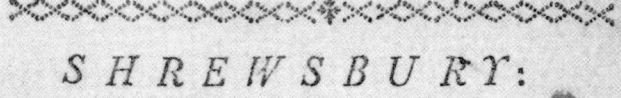

SHREWSBURY:
Printed by W. WILLIAMS.

FREEMAN, S.

270 The farrier's vade mecum; or, gentleman's pocket companion: a compendious treatise on the practice of horse medicine ... / by S. Freeman. — London: Printed for J. Wheble ..., 1772. — [4], xi, [21], 192, [4]p, [1] folded leaf of plates: ill; 17cm (12mo)
Illustration: page 77

FREEMAN, Strickland

271 Observations on the mechanism of the horse's foot: its natural spring explained, and a mode of shoeing recommended ... / by Strickland Freeman, esq. — London: Printed by W. Bulmer and Co. for the author, and sold by G. Nicol ..., 1796. — [4], viii, 107, [32]p, 16, 16 leaves of plates: ill (some col.); 29cm (4to)
Each of 16 plates in both colour and outline
With author's bookplate

272 **FULL INSTRUCTIONS FOR COUNTRY GENTLEMEN, FARMERS, GRASIERS, FARRIERS, CARRIERS, SPORTSMEN, &C.**: being a very curious collection of well-experienced observations and receipts for the cure of most common distempers ... / by a Society of Country Gentlemen, Farmers, Graziers, Sportsmen, &c. — London: Printed and sold by E. Owen ... and T. Astley ..., 1732. — [4], 90, [6]p; 19cm (8vo)

G.L.

273 The gentleman's new jockey: or, farrier's approved guide: containing the exactest rules and methods for breeding and managing horses ... — London: Printed by W.W. for Nicholas Boddington ..., 1687. — [24], 214p: ill; 15cm (12mo)
Preface signed: G.L.
Imperfect: frontispiece missing

274 The gentleman's new jockey: or, farrier's approved guide: containing the exactest rules and methods for breeding and managing horses ... — The third edition, with large additions. — London: Printed by W. Onley, for Nicholas Boddington ..., 1696. — [20], 184p: ill; 16cm (12mo)
Preface signed: G.L.
Imperfect: frontispiece missing

275 The gentleman's new jockey: or, farrier's approved guide: containing the exactest rules and methods for breeding and managing horses ... — The seventh edition, with large additions. — London: Printed for M. Boddington ..., 1721. — [20], 196p: ill; 16cm (12mo)
Preface signed: G.L.
Imperfect: frontispiece missing?

276 **GADSDEN'S PATENT VETERINARY MEDICAL CASE.** — Philadelphia: J.W. Gadsden, 1872. — 39p: ill; 15cm

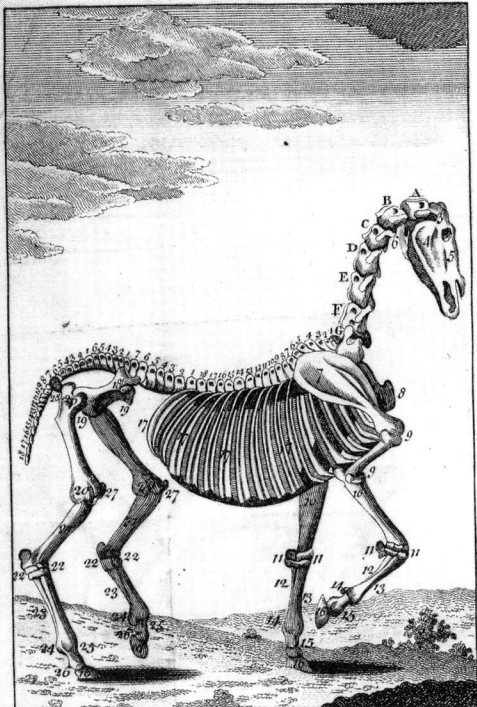

THE
FARRIER's
VADE MECUM;
OR,
Gentleman's Pocket Companion:
A
COMPENDIOUS TREATISE
ON THE
Practice of Horse Medicine, or the Art of Farriery.

To comprise every thing which is really useful.

The Disorders by which that noble Animal the Horse is liable to be affected are critically defined, their Causes ascertained; and Methods of radical and absolute Cure are here prescribed.

To which are added,

SOME THOUGHTS ON THE PLAGUE

And other Disorders in Horned Cattle;

And rendered compleat by

An APPENDIX,

Exhibiting an Account of the Drugs required in Practice, as to their Nature, Qualities and Medicinal Virtues. With a valuable Prescription for the Epidemical Disorder that sometimes rages in this and other Climates.

By S. FREEMAN.

LONDON:
Printed for J. Wheble, No. 24, Pater-noster Row.
M DCC LXXII.

GAMGEE, John, 1831-1894

277 Dairy stock: its selection, diseases, and produce, with a description of the Brittany breed / by John Gamgee. — Edinburgh: T.C. Jack, 1861. — [4], viii, 316p, [3] leaves of plates: ill; 18cm

278 Our domestic animals in health and disease / by John Gamgee. — Edinburgh: Maclachlan & Stewart; London: Simpkin, Marshall, & Co., 1875. — 2v (vi, [4], 640; xvi, 631p): ill; 19cm

GAMGEE, Joseph, 1801-1895

279 Plain rules for the stable / by Professor Gamgee, senr. and John Gamgee. — 2nd ed. rev. and enl. — London: F. Warne and Co., 1866. — 72p: ill; 17cm

280 The **GENTLEMAN FARRIER**: containing instructions for the choice, and directions in the management of horses ... / published by the direction of a person of quality. — London: Printed for F. Cogan ... and H. Lintot ..., 1732. — [18], 137, [13]p; 17cm (12mo)

281 The **GENTLEMAN FARRIER**: containing instructions for the choice, and directions in the management of horses ... / published by the direction of a person of quality. — The second edition. — London: Printed for F. Cogan ... and H. Lintot ..., 1732. — [18], 137, [13]p; 17cm (12mo)

282 The **GENTLEMAN OR TRAVELLER'S POCKET-FARRIER**: and horseman's tutor ... — Northampton: [s.n.], 1732. — vi, [7]-88p; 13cm (16mo)
Illustration: page 79

GEYELIN, George Kennedy

283 Poultry breeding in a commercial point of view: as carried out by the National Poultry Company ... / by Geo. Kennedy Geyelin. — London: Simpkin & Marshall, 1865. — 95p, [1] leaf of plates: ill; 22cm

GIBSON, William, 1680?-1750

284 The farriers dispensatory: in three parts ... / by W. Gibson. — London: Printed for W. Taylor ..., 1721. — [12], 306, [18]p; 21cm (8vo)

285 The farrier's dispensatory: in three parts ... / by W. Gibson. — The second edition corrected. — London: Printed for J. Osborn and T. Longman ..., 1726. — [11], 306, [18], 8p; 20cm (8vo)

286 The farrier's dispensatory: in three parts ... / by W. Gibson. — The fifth edition, corrected. — London: Printed for T. Longman ..., 1741. — [11], 306, [18]p; 20cm (8vo)
The first (1721) edition of The farriers dispensatory has, A1, title; A2, Dedication; A3-A6, Preface. In subsequent editions an advertisement leaf, which is A1, is introduced before the title which becomes A2; A3, Dedication is then erroneously signatured A2; Preface commences on A4. This error gives a false impression that copies lack leaf A3

THE
GENTLEMAN or TRAVELLER's
Pocket-Farrier,
AND
Horseman's Tutor.

DIRECTING

How a HORSE should be used on a Journey.

TOGETHER WITH

Proper REMEDIES for such Misfortunes as may befal him on the Road. Likewise some useful Directions towards the Chusing and Buying of HORSES. As also, Certain Rules to know the Age of any HORSE; with Instructions whereby the Buyer may (*if carefully observ'd*) prevent being impos'd upon (*as they too frequently are*) by Jockies and Dealers.

To which is added,

Several curious and very necessary Observations, and the most proper and valuable Receipts from the best Authors: Together with a true Description of the Farcin and Glanders, worthy to be taken Notice of by all Lovers of Horses.

―――― *Queis gratior usus Equorum*
Nocturna versate manu, versate diurnâ.

Northampton, Printed in the Year 1732.

287 The farriers new guide: containing first, the anatomy of a horse ... secondly, an account of all the diseases ... / by W. Gibson. — London: Printed for William Taylor ..., 1720. — xii, viii, 125, [3], 303, [1]p, [8] leaves of plates (1 folded): ill; 20cm (8vo)

288 The farrier's new guide: containing, first, the anatomy of a horse ... / by W. Gibson. — The ninth edition corrected. — London: Printed for T. Longman ..., 1738. — [16], 109, [1] (blank), [2], 260, [2]p, [8] leaves of plates (1 folded): ill; 20cm (8vo)
The engraved plates in The farrier's new guide consist of a folded frontispiece, A table of diseases, usually bound in to face the general title; and seven anatomical plates evidently redrawn from Snape (573), throughout the first part: there are no plates in the second part
Illustration: page 81

289 A new treatise on the diseases of horses: wherein what is necessary to the knowledge of a horse ... are fully discussed ... / by William Gibson ... — London: Printed for A. Millar ..., 1751. — [12], 464, [12]p, [1], XXXI leaves of plates: ill; 30cm (4to)
Illustration: page 17

290 A new treatise on the diseases of horses: wherein what is necessary to the knowledge of a horse, the cure of his diseases, and other matters relating to that subject, are fully discussed ... / by William Gibson ... — The second edition, corrected. — London: Printed for A. Millar ..., 1754. — 2v ([12], 388p, [22] leaves of plates; [2], 428, [18]p, [10] leaves of plates): ill; 21cm (8vo)

291 [New treatise on the diseases of horses. Selections] Mr. Gibson's short practical method of cure for horses: extracted from his New treatise on their diseases ... / by his son William Gibson. — London: Printed for A. Millar ..., 1755. — [12], 249, [11]p, [10] leaves of plates: ill; 19cm (8vo)
The 32 copper plates announced on the title of the first (1751) 4to edition of A new treatise ... consist of a frontispiece and 31 numbered plates bound together at the end of the volume. The 31 plates were re-engraved for the second (1754) edition in two volumes 8vo. The abridged work by William Gibson (son) (1755) contains only the ten plates numbered 22 to 31 from the 1754 edition

292 The true method of dieting horses: containing many curious and useful observations concerning their marks, colour and external shape ... / by W. Gibson. — London: Printed for W. Taylor ..., 1721. — [4], viij, iv, [4], 236, vij, [1] (blank), 16p; 20cm (8vo)

293 The true method of dieting horses: containing many curious and useful observations concerning their marks, colour and external shape ... / by W. Gibson. — The third edition, corrected. — London: Printed for John Osborn and Tho. Longman ..., 1731. — [2], iv, iv, [4], 236, vjp; 20cm (8vo)

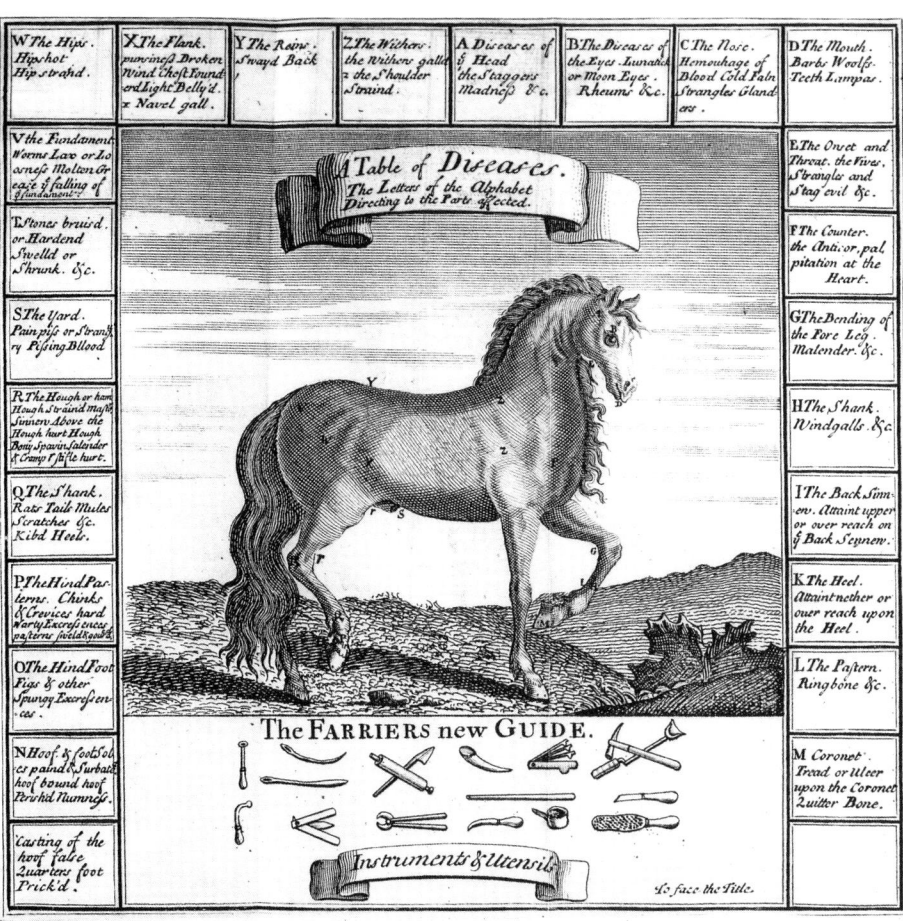

GILBEY, Sir Walter, 1831-1914

294 Pig in health: and how to avoid swine-fever / by Sir Walter Gilbey, Bart. — 2nd ed. — [London]: Vinton & Co., 1910. — [4], 38p, [3] leaves of plates: ill; 22cm

295 Poultry-keeping on farms and small holdings / by Sir Walter Gilbey, Bart. — London: Vinton & Co., 1904. — vi, 38p, [6] leaves of plates: ill; 22cm

GIRARD, F. N. (François Narcisse), 1796-1825

296 A treatise on the teeth of the horse: shewing its age ... / translated from the French of M. Girard by T. Irwin Ganly. — London: Sherwood, Gilbert, and Piper, 1829. — viii, 75p, II leaves of plates: col.ill.; 19cm (12mo)

GLYNN, Ernest, d. 1929

297 The study of disease in the domesticated animals, its importance to the community, with a plea for an animal hospital: an inaugural lecture ... University of Liverpool ... 1913 / by Ernest Glynn. — Liverpool: University Press of Liverpool, 1913. — 40p; 22cm
Presentation copy (inscription)

GRAHAM, Thomas C.

298 The cow and sheep doctor: describing the proper treatment ... / by Thomas C. Graham. — Dublin: W. Leckie, 1852. — 62p; 21cm

GRAY, D. J. Thomson

299 Poultry ailments and their treatment: for the use of amateurs / by D.J. Thomson Gray. — Dundee: J.P. Mathew; London: L. Upcott Gill, 1885. — 56p: ill; 18cm

GRAY, Thomas de
see DE GRAY, Thomas

GRIFFITHS, William

300 A practical treatise on farriery: deduced from the experience of above forty years ... / by William Griffiths .... — Wrexham: Printed by R. Marsh, 1784. — [4], iii, [1], 184, [12]p, [1] leaf of plates: ill; 25cm (4to)
Subscribers names: p.[5-12]
"The following remarkable nostrum ..." pasted on p.[4] at the end

301 A practical treatise on farriery: deduced from the experience of above fifty years ... / by William Griffiths ... — Wrexham: Printed by J. Marsh at the Druid Press, 1795. — [4], iii, [1], 184, [14]p, [2] leaves of plates: ill, port; 26cm (4to)

A list of the subscribers: p.[11-14]
The first edition of A practical treatise on farriery (in which the Dedication is dated 13th November 1784) has a frontispiece by H. Bunbury also dated 1784. The second edition (1795) has the same frontispiece and in addition an engraved portrait of Griffiths bound between A2 and A3. Smith (II, 145) mentions the high standard of production of this work; surviving copies are invariably found in bindings of luxurious full tree calf with gilt decorated spines and labels with the lettering within a fancy gilt lozenge design – evidently a quality publisher's binding in which all copies were issued

GRISONE, Federico

302 Gli ordini di cavalcare / di Federigo Grisone, gentil'huomo napoletano. — In Napoli: Appresso Giouan Paulo Suganappo, 1550. — [2], CXXIIII, [30] leaves: ill; 20cm (4to)
Imprint from colophon
Leaves 117-120 foliated with arabic numerals
The final [30] leaves (AAA_1 to HHH_2) contain 50 whole-page woodcuts of horse bits

303 Ordini di cavalcare: et modi di conoscere le nature de cavalli ... / composti dal Sig. Federico Grisone napolitano. — [S.l.: s.n.], 1561. — 110, [26] leaves: ill; 16cm (8vo)
The final [26] leaves (O_7 to R_8) contain 50 whole-page woodcuts of horse bits

304 Ordini di cavalcare: et modi di conoscere le nature de'caualli ... / del sig. Federico Grisone, gentil'huomo napolitano; aggiungeuisi vna Scielta di notabili auuertimenti ... — Di nuouo migliorati ... — In Venetia: Appresso gli heredi di Luigi Valuassori, & Gio. Domenico Micheli, 1584. — [12], 163, [1], 71, [12]p: ill; 22cm (4to)
Scielta has separate t.p. and pagination
Pages 114 to 163 (H_1 verso to K_{10}) contain 50 whole-page woodcuts of horse bits
Illustration: page 84

GUÉRINIÈRE, François Robichon de la
see LA GUÉRINIÈRE, François Robichon de, d.1751

GUILLET DE SAINT-GEORGE, Georges, 1625?-1705
305 [Les arts de l'homme d'épée. English] The gentleman's dictionary: in three parts. Viz. I. The art of riding the great horse ... II. The military art ... III. The art of navigation ... each part done alphabetically, from the sixteenth edition of the original French / published by the Sieur Guillet ... — London: Printed for H. Bonwicke ... [and 4 others], 1705. — [384]p, [3] folded leaves of plates: ill; 18cm (8vo)

GUNNING, Thomas
306 A short treatise on the late distemper among horned cattle / by Thomas Gunning. — Sligo: J.E. Thacker, 1845. — 15p; 16cm (8vo)

H., J.
see HALFPENNY, John

INFERMITA', CHE SOGLIONO MOLESTARE I CAVALLI.

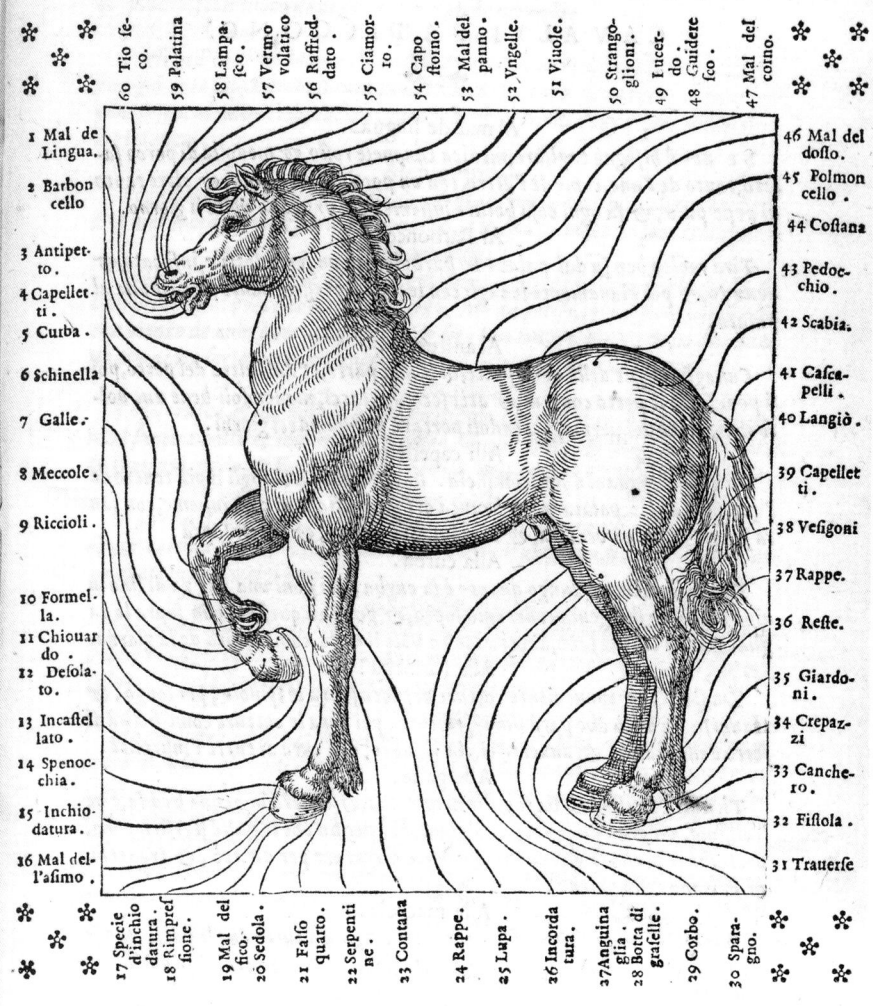

HALFPENNY, John

307 The gentleman's jocky, and approved farrier: instructing, in the natures, causes, and cures of all diseases incident to horses ... / with divers other curiosities collected by the long practice, experience and pains of J.H. esquire ... [et al.]. — London: Printed for Hen. Twyford ... and Nath. Brook ..., 1671. — [16], 300, [4]p, [1] folded leaf of plates: ill; 17cm (8vo)
J.H. is John Halfpenny
Reference: Wing (2nd ed.) H283
Illustration: page 86

308 The gentleman's jockey, and approved farrier: instructing in the natures, causes, and cures of all diseases incident to horses ... / with divers other curiosities, collected by the long practice, experience, and pains of J.H. esq. ... [et al.]. — The eighth edition with additions. — London: Printed for H.T. and O.B. and sold by Timothy Goodwin ..., 1687. — [16], 271, [1]p, [1] folded leaf of plates: ill; 18cm (8vo)
J.H. is John Halfpenny

HALSE, Edward

309 The liver-fluke and the rot in sheep: a prize essay / by Edward Halse. — London: E. Stanford, 1887. — 62p, [1] folded leaf of plates: ill; 19cm

HANGER, George, 1751?-1824

310 General George Hanger to all sportsmen, farmers, and gamekeepers: above thirty years' practice in horses and dogs ... — A new edition. — London: Printed for J.J. Stockdale, [1816?]. — [3]-226p, [1] folded leaf of plates: ill; 22cm (8vo)

HARLEY, William, d. 1830

311 The Harleian dairy system: and an account of the various methods of dairy husbandry pursued by the Dutch ... / by William Harley. — London: J. Ridgway, 1829. — xxxvi, 288p, [6] leaves of plates (some folded): ill, plans, port; 22cm (8vo)

HARRISON, Edward, 1766-1838

312 On the rot in sheep / by Edward Harrison ... — Bury, St. Edmund's: J. Rackham ..., 1803. — 40p; 21cm (8vo)
Presentation copy (inscription)

HASLAM, James

313 Veterinary chart: or a practical treatise on the diseases of the horse: their causes, symptoms, and treatment ... / by James Haslam. — Manchester: Printed by Ratcliffe and Co., [18--]. — 34p; 22cm (8vo)

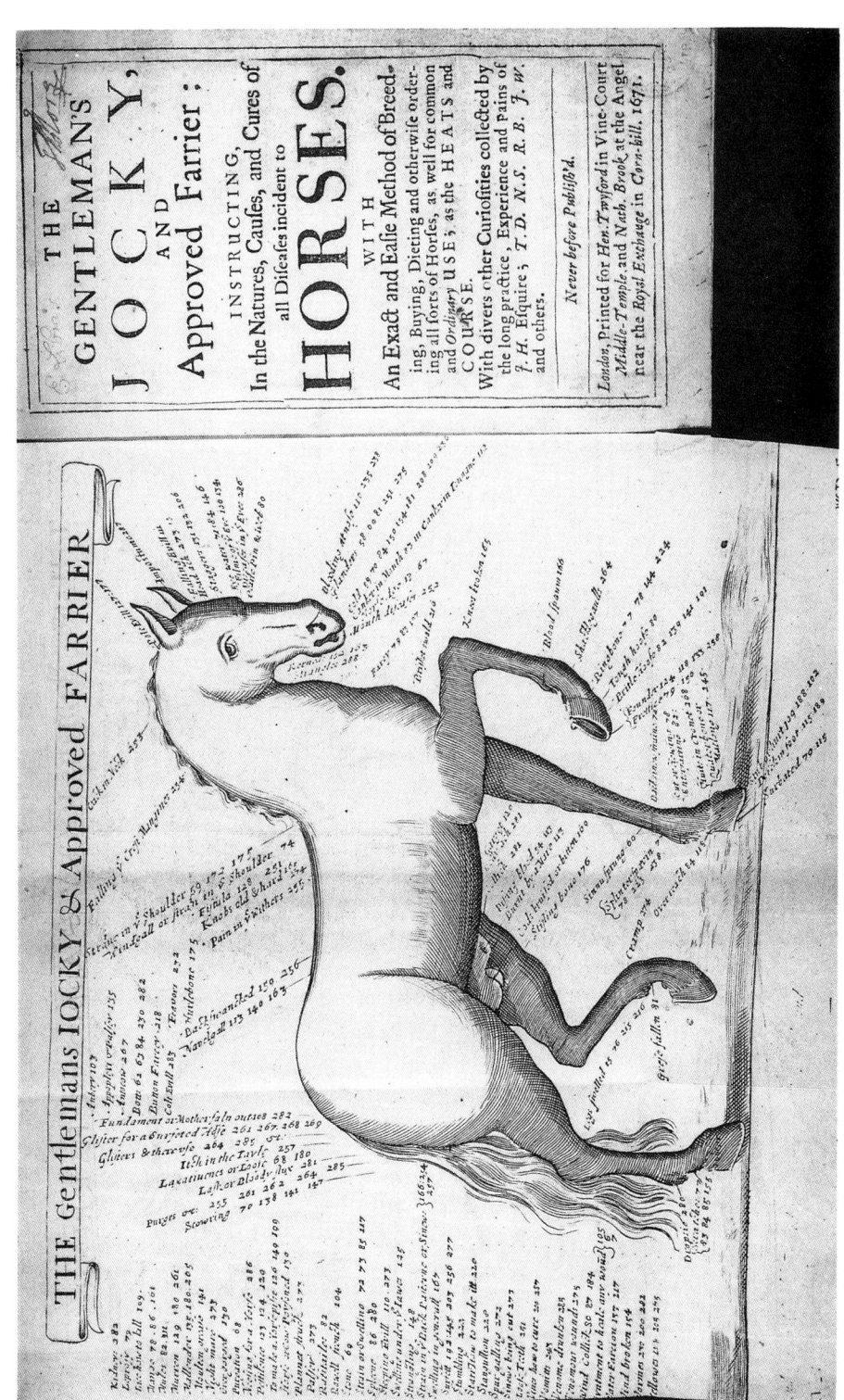

Halfpenny 1671 (307)

HASTFER, Frederic W., 1722-1762

314 [Utförlig och omständelig underrättelse om fullgoda fårs ans och skjötsel. French] Instruction sur la manière d'élever et de perfectionner les bestes à laine / composée en suédois par Frederic W. Hastfer ; mise en françois par M. ***. — A Paris: Chez Guillyn ...; et à Dijon: Chez François Desventes, 1756. — xliv, 178, [4], 238, [2]p; 17cm (12mo)
Translated by Claude Carlier
Pt.2 has separate t.p. and pagination

315 The **HAY & CATTLE MEASURER**: a series of tables ... — London: Blackie and Son, 1860. — 124p, [1] leaf of plates: ill; 18cm

HAYCOCK, W. (William), 1818-1872

316 On the education and training of the veterinary pupil: the present state of veterinary medicine ... / by W. Haycock. — London: Printed by J.E. Adlard, 1866. — 15p; 21cm
Presidential address to the Lancashire Veterinary Medical Association, Jan. 10, 1866 (Smith, IV, 115 – '... probably his finest literary effort.')

HAYWOOD, William, 1821-1894

317 Report to the Honourable the Commissioners of Sewers of the City of London on the accidents to horses on carriageway pavements / by William Haywood. — London: Charles Skipper & East, printers, 1873. — 145p (some folded); 21cm
Presentation copy (inscription)
Imperfect: lacking p.145

HEARSON, Charles E.

318 The problem solved: a practical treatise on artificial incubation and chicken rearing / by Chas. E. Hearson. — 27th ed. — London: Spratt's Patent, [1910?]. — 96p: ill; 21cm

HENDERSON, Andrew

319 The practical grazier; or, a treatise on the proper selection and management of live stock ... / by Andrew Henderson. — Edinburgh: Oliver & Boyd, 1826. — xxvii, 446p, [1], XIII leaves of plates: ill, plans; 22cm (8vo)
Subscribers: p.[443]-446

HENDERSON, Robert

320 A treatise on the breeding of swine: and curing of bacon; with hints on agricultural subjects / by Robert Henderson ... — Leith: Printed and sold by Archibald Allardice ... [and 10 others], 1811. — viii, 118p, [2] leaves of plates: ill, plan; 22cm (8vo)

321 A treatise on the breeding of swine: and curing of bacon; with hints on agricultural subjects / by Robert Henderson ... — Second edition, enlarged and improved. — Leith: Printed and sold by Archibald Allardice ... [and 4 others], 1814. — viii, 139p, [2] leaves of plates: ill, plan; 23cm (8vo)

(cont.)

Newspaper cutting pasted in
Both editions of Henderson's Treatise contain two engraved plates, one of a large curly-coated pig, the other a farm plan for a swine yard

HERESBACH, Conrad, 1496-1576

322 [Rei rusticae libri quatuor. English] Foure bookes of husbandrie / collected by M. Conradus Heresbachius ...; newly Englished, and increased by Barnabe Googe, esquire. — At London: Printed for Iohn Wight, 1586. — [12], 193, [1] leaves: ill, coat of arms; 19cm (4to)

323 [Rei rusticae libri quatuor. English] Foure bookes of husbandry / collected by M. Conradus Heresbachius ...; newly Englished, and encreased by Barnaby Googe, esquire. — London: Printed by Tho. Wight, 1601. — [10], 183, [1] leaves: coat of arms; 18cm (4to)

324 [Rei rusticae libri quatuor. English] The whole art and trade of husbandry: contained in foure bookes ... / enlarged by Barnaby Googe, esquire. — London: Printed by T.S. for Richard More ..., 1614. — [11], 183 leaves; 18cm (4to)
By Conrad Heresbach

325 [Rei rusticae libri quatuor. English] The whole art of husbandry: contained in foure bookes ... / first written by Conrade Heresbatch, a learned nobleman; then translated by Barnaby Googe esquire; and now renewed, corrected, enlarged ... by Captaine Gervase Markham. — London: Printed by T.C. for Richard More ..., 1631. — [8], 385, [1]p; 19cm (4to)

HICKEY, William
see DOYLE, Martin

HILL, Caleb

326 The origin of the epidemic which has affected vegetation & cattle since the famine in Ireland ... / by Caleb Hill. — Axbridge: Oliver & Son, [1870]. — 20p; 21cm

HILL, J. Woodroffe (John Woodroffe), d. 1909

327 The diseases of poultry: their causes, symptoms and treatment. A practical guide book for the use of amateurs / by J. Woodroffe Hill. — London: Published at the office of "Poultry", [1884]. — 108, xxip; 19cm

HILLYARD, C. (Clark)

328 Practical farming and grazing: with observations on the breeding and feeding of sheep and cattle ... / by C. Hillyard. — 3rd ed. — Northampton: T.E. Dicey, 1840. — viii, 168, 3, 12, [4]p, [1] leaf of plates: ill; 22cm (12mo)

HINDS, John

329 Conversations on conditioning. The grooms' oracle, and pocket stable-directory: in which the management of horses ... are considered ... / John Hinds. — 2nd ed. — London: Printed for the author, 1830. — xii, 298, [2]p, [1] folded leaf of plates: col.ill; 20cm (12mo)

330 Multum in parvo: a compendious pocket-manual of the veterinary art ... / by John Hinds and others. — London: Sherwood, Gilbert & Piper, 1832. — x, [11]-216p, [1] folded leaf of plates: ill; 17cm (12mo)
Smith (IV, 8-9) claims that John Hinds was the pseudonym of Badcock the publisher

[HIPPIATRICA]

331 Ton 'ippiatrikon biblia duo = Veterinariae medicinae libri duo / a Ioanne Ruellio Suessionensi olim quidem Latinitate donati, nunc uero ijdem sua, hoc est Graeca, lingua primum in lucem aediti. — Basileae: Apud Ioan. Valderum, 1537. — [12], 307p; 23cm (4to)
Greek title transliterated
Edited by Simon Grynaeus
References: Adams V618; Wellcome (pre-1641) 5619
Bound with: Pub. Vegetii ... Mulomedicina. — Basileae: Per Petrum Pernam, 1574

332 Opera della medicina de cavalli / composta da diversi antichi scrittori, et a commune utilita, di Greco in buona lingua volgare ridotta. — In Venetia: [Michele Tramezino], 1543. — 207, [5] leaves; 16cm (8vo)
Colophon reads: Stampata in Vineggia per Michele Tramezino

333 Opera della medicina de cavalli: composta da diuersi antichi scrittori; et a commune utilita di Greco in buona lingua uolgare ridotta. — Nuouamente da molti errori corretta, & ristampata. — In Venetia: Appresso P. Gironimo Giglio, e compagni, 1559. — 184, [6] leaves; 15cm (8vo)

HOGG, James, 1770-1835

334 The shepherd's guide: being a practical treatise ... / by James Hogg ... — Edinburgh: Printed by J. Ballantyne and Co. for Archibald Constable and Co. ... and John Murray ... London, 1807. — vi, 338, [24]p; 23cm (8vo)

HOLLINSHEAD, John

335 Hints to country gentlemen and farmers on the importance of using salt as a general manure / by John Hollinshead, esq. Chorley. — The second edition. — Blackburn: Printed by Hemingway and Crook, 1800. — 60p; 18cm (8vo)
Disbound

HOLLOWAY, Alfred

336 Practical poultry farming: on-business-lines right down-to-date. — 3rd ed. — Bletchley: Prof. Holloway & Sons, [1907]. — 101+p: ill; 19cm

HORNE, T. H. (Thomas Hartwell), 1780-1862

337 The complete grazier; or, farmer and cattle-dealer's assistant: comprising instructions for the buying, breeding ... / by a Lincolnshire grazier, assisted by communications from several Yorkshire, Leicester, & Norfolk farmers. — London: Printed for B. Crosby ... and sold by S. and J. Ridge ... [and 18 others], 1805. — [6], 510p, [4] leaves of plates (1 folded): ill, plans; 22cm (8vo)
By T.H. Horne
References: Perkins, p.64; Southampton, 823

338 The complete grazier; or farmer's and cattle-breeder and dealer's assistant: comprising instructions for the buying, breeding ... / by a Lincolnshire grazier: assisted by communications from several Yorkshire, Leicester, and Norfolk farmers. — Fourth edition. Revised, corrected, enlarged, and greatly improved. — London: Printed for Baldwin, Cradock, and Joy ..., 1816. — [16], 592p, 5 leaves of plates: ill, plans; 22cm (8vo)
By T.H. Horne
References: Perkins, p.64; Southampton, 824

339 The **HORSE OWNER'S HANDY NOTE BOOK**: or, common diseases of horses and other animals, with their remedies. With which is incorporated a descriptive list of Harvey's great remedies ... — 11th ed. — Dublin: Harvey & Co., 1892. — 96p: ill; 16cm

340 The **HORSEMAN AND TRAVELLER'S PERFECT DIRECTOR, AND POCKET FARRIER**: shewing, in every case, what methods ought to be used ... — London: Printed for J. Hazard ... and W. Bickerton ..., [17--]. — vi, [7]-88, [8]p; 13cm (16mo)
Imperfect: last 2 leaves missing
A blatant plagiarism of Capt. William Burdon's The gentleman's pocket-farrier; shewing, how to use your horse on a journey ... (1730, et seq) (117)
Illustration: page 91

341 **HORSES, CATTLE, SHEEP, PIGS, DOGS, CATS, POULTRY, BIRDS, ETC.**: how to keep them well and treat them when they are ill / by White Horse. — Glasgow: D. Bryce & Son, 1912. — 267, [1]p: ill; 12cm
Produced to advertise Mackie's White Horse whisky

342 **HORSES, DOGS, BIRDS, CATTLE**: accidents and ailments, first aid. — Slough: Elliman, Sons and Co., [1902]. — 32, [1]p: ill; 16cm
Reduced facsimile of the first 32p of: The uses of Elliman's embrocation — 3rd ed.

343 **HOW MY HUNTER WAS LAMED.** — [Slough: Elliman, Sons and Co., 1886?]. — 32p: ill; 22cm

THE
HORSEMAN and TRAVELLER'S
Perfect Director,
AND
Pocket Farrier.

Shewing, in every Cafe,
What METHODS ought to be ufed
on any Misfortunes falling on the Road, or
in the Stable. Likewife ufeful and neceffary
Inftructions for the Choice and Buying of
HORSES; with unerring Rules to know
the Age; which, if regularly minded, the
Purchafer will put it out of the Power of
Jockeys and Dealers vilely to cheat and im-
pofe on them (*as is too frequently practifed.*)
To which are fubjoin'd,
Many curious and worthy Obfervations, fit
to be taken Notice of by all fuch as love or keep Horfes;
with the moft experienced and proper Receipts, as well
from the beft Authors as Practice; and a true Defcrip-
tion, with the Cure, of the Cholick, Farcin, Staggers,
and the Glanders, in many Stations; with a compeat
Alphabetical INDEX for the readier finding any thing
therein contain'd.

LONDON: Printed for J. HAZARD near *Stationers-Hall*, and
W. BICKERTON, at Lord *Bacon*'s Head, without *Temple-Bar*.

HUGHES, Charles
344 The compleat horseman; or, the art of riding made easy: illustrated by rules drawn from nature ... / by Charles Hughes ... — London: Printed for F. Newbery ... and sold at Hughes's Riding-School, [1772]. — 61p, [6] leaves of plates: ill; 18cm (12mo)
Two copies: one imperfect, bound with: The husbandman's companion; and gentleman's amusement

HUNT, C. H. (Charles Henry)
345 A practical treatise on the Merino and Anglo-Merino breeds of sheep: in which the advantages to the farmer and grazier, peculiar to these breeds, are clearly demonstrated / by an experienced breeder. — London: Printed for W. Plant Piercy ... by J.M'Creery ..., 1809. — viii, 198, [2], 4p; 23cm (8vo)
By C.H. Hunt

HUNTER, J. (James)
346 A complete dictionary of farriery & horsemanship: containing the art of farriery ... / the whole compiled from the best authors, by J. Hunter ... — Dublin: Printed for P. Wogan, P. Byrne, J. Rice, and J. Moore, 1796. — vii, [342]p; 21cm (8vo)

347 A complete dictionary of farriery & horsemanship: containing the art of farriery ... / the whole compiled from the best authors, by J. Hunter ... — Birmingham: Printed & sold by T. Pearson; sold also by R. Baldwin & L.B. Seeley ... London, 1796. — v, [300]p, [1] leaf of plates: ill; 23cm (8vo)

HUNTER, John, 1728-1793
348 Account of the free martin / by John Hunter ... — [London: Royal Society, 1779]. — p.279-293; 22cm
Extracted from: Philosophical transactions, vol.69

349 The **HUSBANDMAN'S COMPANION;** and gentleman's amusement. — [S.l.: s.n., 17--]. — 92p; 17cm (12mo)
Imperfect. Lacks t.p.and all before B1. Bound with: The compleat horseman / by Charles Hughes. — London: F. Newbery, [1772]

350 The **HUSBANDMAN'S JEWEL**: directing how to improve land ... — London: Printed for G. Conyers ..., [1720?]. — 52p: ill; 15cm (12mo)
Bound with: The compleat husbandman / by G. Markham.— London: G. Conyers, 1707

HUXTABLE, A. (Anthony), 1808-1883
351 A lecture on the science and application of manures: with an appendix / by A. Huxtable. — 5th ed. — London: J. Ridgway, 1847. — 32p; 22cm (8vo)
Bound with: High farming / by James Caird. — 5th ed. — Edinburgh: W. Blackwood and Sons, 1849

INDUS

352 A view of the policy of Sir George Barlow: as exhibited in the acts of the Madras government ... / by Indus. — London: Printed by Joyce Gold ... for J. Ridgway ..., 1810. — viii, 100, [4]p; 22cm (8vo)
Bound with: Facts and observations relative to sheep, wool, ploughs, and oxen / by John, Lord Somerville. — London: W. Miller, 1803

J.B.
see BLAGRAVE, Joseph, 1610-1682

J.H.
see HALFPENNY, John

J.L.R.

353 Traité des oiseaux de basse-cour et du lapin domestique / par J.L.R. — Paris: Audot, 1823. — [4], 262, 24p, 2 leaves of plates; 18cm (8vo)

J.W.
see WORLIDGE, John

JARDINE, Sir William, 1800-1874

354 The natural history of Gallinaceous birds. Vol.1 / by Sir William Jardine; with memoir of Aristotle by Andrew Crichton. — Edinburgh: W.H. Lizars; London: S. Highley; Dublin: W. Curry, 1836. — 232p, [2], 29 leaves of plates: col.ill, port; 17cm (8vo). — (The naturalist's library. Ornithology; vol.3: Gallinaceous birds)
Added engraved t.p.

355 The natural history of game-birds / by Sir William Jardine. — Edinburgh: W.H. Lizars; London: S. Highley; Dublin: W. Curry, 1834. — [iii]-xi, [1] blank, [17]-197p, [2], 30 leaves of plates: col.ill, port; 17cm (8vo). — (The naturalist's library. Ornithology; vol.4: Gallinaceous birds, part 2: Game-birds)
Added engraved t.p.

JEFFRAY, James, 1759-1848

356 An address to the public, on the present state of farriery / by James Jeffray ... — Edinburgh: [s.n.], 1786. — [6], 12p; 25cm (4to)
Not known to Smith. Jeffray is described as Late President of the Royal Medical Society, Edinburgh &c, and Farrier to His Royal Highness The Prince of Wales for Scotland. He emphasises the need in Britain for a Veterinary School on the lines of those in Lyons and Paris. He offers – if he is given financial support – to study at the continental schools and to prepare lectures for presentation at a similar School that would be established in Britain. This coincides with the movement initiated by the Odiham Agricultural Society in 1785 which led eventually to the establishment of the London Veterinary College in 1791. Jeffray's offer and proposals do not appear to have received support
Illustration: page 94

AN ADDRESS

TO THE

PUBLIC,

ON THE

PRESENT STATE OF FARRIERY.

BY *JAMES JEFFRAY*, A. M.

LATE PRESIDENT OF THE ROYAL MEDICAL SOCIETY, EDINBURGH, &c.
AND FARRIER TO HIS ROYAL HIGHNESS THE PRINCE OF WALES
FOR SCOTLAND.

[*DEDICATED, BY PERMISSION, TO HIS ROYAL HIGHNESS.*]

EDINBURGH. 1786.

JOHNSON, Cuthbert W. (Cuthbert William), 1799-1878
357 The farmers' medical dictionary: for the diseases of animals / by Cuthbert W. Johnson. — London: J. Ridgway, 1845. — 279p; 18cm (12mo)

358 The farmers' medical dictionary: for the diseases of animals / by Cuthbert W. Johnson. — 2nd ed. — London: J. Ridgway, [18--]. — 279p; 18cm
Not included in the list of Johnson's works which Fussell (III, 128) considered to be complete

359 The modern dairy and cowkeeper / by Cuthbert W. Johnson. — London: J. Ridgway, 1850. — 119p, [4] leaves of plates: ill; 19cm (12mo)

JOHNSON, G. M. T. (George Munn Tracy), b.1838
360 Practical poultry keeping: as I understand it / G.M.T. Johnson. — 5th ed. — Binghamton, N.Y.: G.M.T. Johnson, 1886. — 120p, [2] col. leaves of plates: ill; 19cm
Two copies, one in publisher's paper wrappers

JOYCE MAYDWELL AND CO.
361 Graziers, farmers & owners of live stock: sportsmen, trainers & horsekeepers may rely upon ... Maydwell's Driffield oils ... / prepared and sold by Joyce Maydwell & Co. — London: W. Hanson, medical printer, [18--]. — [4]p: ill; 18cm
Cover title

KAUSCH, J. J. (Johann Joseph), 1751-1825
362 Kameralprincipien über Rindviehsterben: für Landesregierungen und angehende Staatswirthe: eine Beilage zu den kameralistischen und staatsarzneilichen Handbüchern ... / von J.J. Kausch. — Berlin: Bei Heinrich August Rottmann, 1793. — XII, 139p, [1] folded leaf of plates: ill; 20cm (8vo)

KENNEDY, L. (Lewis)
363 The present state of the tenancy of land: in the highland and grazing districts in Great Britain ... / L. Kennedy and T.B. Grainger. — London: J. Ridgway, 1829. — xvii, [3], 324p, [1] leaf of plates: ill; 23cm (8vo)

KENNY, E. H.
364 No homestead or stable is complete without E.H. Kenny's preparations: as a guarantee ... dispensed only by R. Roper, chemist, Dunmow. — Bp's Stortford: H. Copley & Co., [1887?]. — [4]p; 12cm

KNOWLSON, John C.
365 The complete cow-leech, or Cattle-doctor: being a treatise on the disorders of horned cattle: with The complete farrier, or horse-doctor ... / by J.C. Knowlson ... — London: Sold by Longman, Hurst, Rees, Orme, Brown and Green ... [and 8 others], 1820. — [2], x, [6], 120, 127, [4]p, [1] leaf of plates: ill; 22cm (8vo)
The 2 pts. have separate title pages and separate pagination

366 The Yorkshire cattle-doctor and farrier ... / John C. Knowlson. — 28th ed. — London; Otley: William Walker & Sons, [189-?]. — xiv, 272p, [2] leaves of plates (1 folded): ill; 22cm

L., G.
The gentleman's new jockey
see G.L.

LA FOSSE, Étienne Guillaume, d.1765
367 Guide du maréchal: ouvrage contenant une connoissance exacte du cheval ... / par M. Lafosse ... — A Paris: Chez Lacombe ..., 1767. — xij, 417, [3]p, [10] folded leaves of plates: ill; 21cm (8vo)
The Avis au relieur calls for 10 plates. These are numbered 1, 2, 4, 4, 5, 3, 6a, 6B, 7, 8

368 [Observations et découvertes faites sur des chevaux. English] Observations and discoveries made upon horses: with a new method of shoeing / by the Sieur La Fosse ... — London: Printed for J. Nourse ..., 1755. — viii [i.e. vii], [1], iv, [5]-120p, 4 folded leaves of plates: ill; 21cm (8vo).
Two copies: one bound with: A dissertation on horses / by William Osmer. — London: T. Waller, 1756

369 [Traité sur le véritable siège de la morve des chevaux. English] A treatise upon the true seat of the glanders in horses: together with the method of cure ... / by Mons. De La Fosse ...; the translation and notes by H. Bracken ... — London: Printed for T. Osborne ..., 1751. — xxiv, 55, [5]p, [1] folded leaf of plates: ill; 17cm (12mo)

LA GUÉRINIÈRE, François Robichon de, d. 1751
370 École de cavalerie: contenant la connoissance, l'instruction, et la conservation du cheval / par M. de la Guérinière ... — A Paris: Chez Jacques Guérin ..., 1736. — 2v ([14], 120 [i.e.320]p, 32 leaves of plates (2 folded); [4], 298p, 2 folded leaves of plates): ill, port; 20cm (8vo)

371 École de cavalerie: contenant la connoissance, l'instruction, et la conservation du cheval / par M. de La Guérinière ... — A Paris: Chez Huart et Moreau ... [and 4 others], 1751. — [8], 318, [10]p, 25 leaves of plates (some folded): ill, plans; 46cm (fol)

372 [École de cavalerie. Italian] La cognizione perfetta del cavallo e della cavallerizza: in tutte le sue parti / ossia il signore della Gueriniere ... Elementi di cavallerizza; tradotti dal francese ... dal Visconte di Milleville ... — In Venezia: Presso Antonio Casali, 1794. — 352p, [9] folded leaves of plates: ill; 15cm (4to)
The 9 folded leaves of plates incorporate 16 plates reduced in size

LAMBERT, J. (James)
373 The country-man's treasure: shewing the nature, causes, and cure of all diseases incident to cattle ... / by J. Lambert, gent. — London: Printed for T. Norris ..., [17--]. — 167, [1]p: ill; 15cm (12mo)
See notes re frontispiece and text under A.S. (4)

LANE, John
374 The principles of English farriery vindicated: containing strictures on the erroneous and long-exploded system, lately revived at the Veterinary College ... / by John Lane ... — [London]: Printed for the author by A. Seale ... and sold by G. Riebau ... [and 6 others], 1800. — [2], 97p; 22cm (8vo)
Lane praises the general standards of farriery in England but is highly critical of the ideas and teaching of the London Veterinary College, and of its Professor Edward Coleman in particular
Illustration: page 98

LASTEYRIE DU SAILLANT, C. P. (Charles Philibert), 1759-1849
375 [Histoire de l'introduction des moutons à laine fine d'Espagne. English] An account of the introduction of Merino sheep: into the different states of Europe, and at the Cape of Good Hope ... / from the French of C.P. Lasteyrie by Benjamin Thompson, with notes by the translator. — London: Printed for John Harding ..., 1810. — vi, [2] (last blank), 248p, 1 leaf of plates: ill; 22cm (8vo)

LAUBENDER, Bernhard, 1764-1815
376 Das ganze der Rindviehpest: oder vollständiger Unterricht die Rindviehpest genau zu erkennen, sicher zu heilen ... / entworfen und dargestellt von Bernhard Laubender ... — Leipzig: Bey Gerhard Fleischer dem Jüngern, 1801. — XVI, 652, [2]p; 18cm (8vo)
Druckfehler: [2]p at the end

LAWES, J. B. (John Bennet), 1814-1900
377 Fifth report of experiments on the feeding of sheep / by J.B. Lawes & J.H. Gilbert. — London: Printed by W. Clowes and Sons, 1861. — 14p; 22cm
From the Journal of the Royal Agricultural Society of England, vol.22, part 1

378 Observations on the recently-introduced manufactured foods for agricultural stock / by J.B. Lawes. — London: Printed by W. Clowes and Sons, 1858: (re-printed by Dunn & Chidgey, 1889). — 8p; 22cm
From the Journal of the Royal Agricultural Society of England, vol.19, part 1

379 Report of experiments on the comparative fattening qualities of different breeds of sheep / by J.B. Lawes. — London: Printed by William Clowes and Sons, 1852. — 34p; 23cm
From the Journal of the Royal Agricultural Society of England, vol.12, part 2

given to Mr Parker by Miss Lane 1804

THE PRINCIPLES OF ENGLISH FARRIERY VINDICATED;

CONTAINING

STRICTURES ON THE ERRONEOUS
AND
LONG-EXPLODED SYSTEM, LATELY REVIVED
AT THE

VETERINARY COLLEGE;

INTERSPERSED WITH
CURSORY REMARKS ON THE SYSTEMS
OF
SOLLEYSELL, DE SAUNIER, DE LA FOSSE, &c. &c

IN WHICH IS FULLY DISPLAYED THE

Superiority of English Farriery

OVER THAT OF FOREIGN NATIONS,

BY JOHN LANE, A. V. P.

LATE OF THE SECOND REGIMENT

OF LIFE-GUARDS.

" Naturam intueamur, hanc sequamur."
Quinct. VIII. 3.

" First follow *Nature*, and your judgement frame
By her just standard, which is still the same;
Unerring *Nature*, still divinely bright,
One clear, unchang'd, and universal light,
Life, force, and beauty, must to all impart,
At once the source, and end, and test of Art."
Pope

PRINTED FOR THE AUTHOR

By A. Seale, No. 34, Goodge-Street, Fitzroy Square, And Sold by G. Riebau, No. 2, Blandford-Street, Manchester Square; Wm. Baynes, Pater–Noster-Row; Lee, Fleet-Street; Bagster, Strand; Cavel, Middle-Row, Holborn; Kirby, Oxford-Street; and Egerton, Charing-Cross.   *Price Four-Shillings*

1800.

LAWRENCE, B.

380 The complete cattle-keeper: or, farmer's and grazier's guide in the choice and management of neat cattle and sheep ... / by B. Lawrence. — London: Dean and Munday, [1831]. — 336p, VI leaves of plates: ill; 17cm (12mo)

LAWRENCE, John, 1753-1839

381 A general treatise on cattle: the ox, the sheep, and the swine ... / by John Lawrence ... — London: Printed for H.D. Symonds ... by C. Whittingham ..., 1805. — [8], 639, [9]p; 21cm (8vo)

382 The history and delineation of the horse: in all his varieties ... / by John Lawrence ... — London: Albion Press: printed for James Cundee ... and John Scott ..., 1809. — iv, [5]-288, [4]p, [15] leaves of plates: ill; 30cm (4to)
Errata: on p.[3]. Additional engr. t.p. and engr. inscription plate
Reference: Huth, p.78

383 Lawrence's agricultural and veterinary works: comprehending a body of useful and practical knowledge ... — London: Printed for Sherwood, Neely, and Jones (successors to Mr. H.D. Symonds), 1810. — 5v; 21cm (8vo)
Imperfect: v.1, 2 and 4 only
Vols. 1 and 2 are a slightly re-arranged re-issue of A philosophical and practical treatise on horses (384) (xix, [1], 624p;xi, [1], 572, [4]p) .Vol. 4 is a re-issue of A general treatise on cattle (381) (xvi, 618, [6]p). The other two volumes consisted of re-issues of The new farmer's calendar; and The modern land steward

384 A philosophical and practical treatise on horses: and on the moral duties of man towards the brute creation / by John Lawrence. — London: Printed for T. Longman ..., 1796-1798. — 2v (viii, 391;viii, 600p); 22cm (8vo)
List of subscribers: v.2, p.[iii]-vi

385 A practical treatise on breeding, rearing and fattening all kinds of domestic poultry, pheasants, pigeons, and rabbits: with an account of the Egyptian method of hatching eggs by artificial heat / by Bonington Moubray. — 2nd ed. — London: Sherwood, Neely and Jones, 1816. — xii, 256p; 18cm (12mo)
Bonington Moubray is the pseud. of John Lawrence

386 A practical treatise on breeding, rearing, and fattening all kinds of domestic poultry, pheasants, pigeons, and rabbits ... / by Bonington Moubray. — 4th ed. with additions. — London: Sherwood, Neely, and Jones, 1822. — xii, 312p, [1] leaf of plates: ill; 20cm (12mo)
Bonington Moubray is the pseud. of John Lawrence
Two copies

387 A practical treatise on breeding, rearing, and fattening all kinds of domestic poultry, pheasants, pigeons, and rabbits: including an interesting account of the Egyptian method of hatching eggs by artificial heat and the author's experiments thereon, also the management of swine, milch cows, and bees and instructions for the private brewery / by Bonington Moubray. — 5th ed. — London: Sherwood, Jones and Co., 1824. — xii, 360p, [1] leaf of plates; 18cm (12mo)
Bonington Moubray is the pseud. of John Lawrence
The 1822 and 1824 editions have a hand-coloured frontispiece plate depicting a Spanish cock and hen; a Suffolk milch cow; and an Oxford dairy pig

388 A treatise on breeding, rearing, and fattening, all kinds of poultry, cows, swine, and other domestic animals / by B. Moubray. — Repr. from the 6th London ed. with ... abridgements, and additions ... / by Thomas G. Fessenden. — Boston: Lilly & Wait: Carter & Hendee, 1832. — 266p: ill; 18cm (12mo)
Title of previous eds.: A practical treatise on breeding, rearing, and fattening all kinds of domestic poultry ...
Bonington Moubray is the pseud. of John Lawrence

389 Moubray's treatise on domestic and ornamental poultry: a practical guide to the history, breeding, rearing, feeding, fattening and general management of fowls and pigeons. — New ed. / rev. and greatly enl. by L.A. Meall; to which is added the diseases of poultry ... by F.R. Horner. — London: Arthur Hall, Virtue and Co., 1854. — viii, 504p, [10] leaves of plates: col.ill; 18cm
Moubray is the pseud. of John Lawrence

The sportsman, farrier and shoeing-smiths, new guide
see SAINBEL, Charles Vial de, 1753-1793

LAWRENCE, Richard
390 An inquiry into the structure & animal oeconomy of the horse: comprehending the diseases to which his limbs and feet are subject, with proper directions for shoeing ... / by Richard Lawrence ... — Birmingham: Printed for the author at T.A. Pearson's ... and sold by Knott & Lloyd ...; [London]: J. Wallis ... and G. Nicol ..., 1801. — xxiv, 212, [30]p, [3], 15 leaves of plates (some folded): ill; 26cm (4to)
List of subscribers: p.[xxi]-xxiv
Reference: Huth, p.67
Smith (III, 107) had only seen the later edition of this title and was not aware of the date of this first edition

LAWSON, A.
391 The farmer's practical instructor: shewing all the latest and most approved methods ... / by A. Lawson. — Newcastle upon Tyne: Mackenzie and Dent, 1827. — 571p, [1], X leaves of plates: ill, port; 22cm (4to)

392 The modern farrier: or, the art of preserving the health and curing the diseases of horses, dogs, oxen, ... / by A. Lawson. — 13th ed. — Newcastle upon Tyne: Mackenzie and Dent, 1829. — 616, viii p, [9] leaves of plates: ill; 22cm (4to)
Added engraved t.p.

LAWSON, S. (Stephen)
393 An essay on the use of mixed and compressed cattle fodder: for feeding and fattening horses, oxen, cows, sheep, hogs or pigs ... / by S. Lawson ... — London: Printed for the author. And sold by Mr. Richardson ... and Mr. Debrett ..., 1797. — [2], ii, [3]-88p; 21cm (8vo)

LAYARD, Daniel Peter, 1721-1802
394 An essay on the nature, causes, and cure of the contagious distemper among the horned cattle in these kingdoms / by Daniel Peter Layard ... — London: Printed for John Rivington ...; Charles Bathurst ...; and Thomas Payne ..., 1757. — xxii, [2], 134, [1]p; 22cm (8vo)
Errata: p.[135]
Presentation copy to the Bishop of Winchester (inscription). Last leaf (K4) used as paste-down

LE CHOYSELAT, Prudent
see PRUDENT LE CHOYSELAT

LEEMING, John
395 Every man his own farrier: or, an introduction to speculative and practical farriery: containing some useful observations on the blood; a sketch of the animal oeconomy ... / by John Leeming ... — [Coventry]: Printed for the author by Messrs. Jopsons ..., 1771. — [4], ii, vi, iv, 200p; 17cm (12mo)
Errata: p.200
An attempt has been made to erase the description Volume I from both the title and the last leaf of this copy of Leeming's work. Apparently unrecorded: not in BL or NUC; not known to Smith or to Huth; not in RVC or RCVS
Illustration: page 102

LEENEY, Harold, b.1852
396 The lambing pen / by Harold Leeney. — London: Printed by Spottiswoode & Co., 1897. — 38p: ill; 22cm
Cover title
From the Journal of the Royal Agricultural Society of England, third series, vol.7, part 4, 1896

LESTER, W. (William)
397 Observations on the utility of cutting hay and straw, and bruising corn, for feeding of animals: arranged and elucidated, not by chemical test but agricultural practice ... / by W. Lester ... — London: Printed by C. Whittingham ... sold by H.D. Symonds ... J. Hatchard ..., 1803. — [4], 34, [1]p, [2] folded leaves of plates: ill; 20cm (8vo)
Disbound

Every Man his own Farrier:

OR, AN

INTRODUCTION

TO

Speculative and Practical Farriery.

CONTAINING

Some useful OBSERVATIONS on the BLOOD;
A Sketch of the ANIMAL ŒCONOMY;
A brief Description of ANATOMY;
An Account of the PULSE;
And Consent of the NERVES.

ALSO,

Particular DIRECTIONS how to apply my
PUBLIC MEDICINES.

To which are prefixed

I. Some useful Observations on FEVERS.
II. Observations on WOUNDS and ULCERS.
III. Observations on LAMENESSES.
With REMARKS on each.

By JOHN LEEMING, FARRIER,

COVENTRY.

Printed for the AUTHOR,
By MESSRS. JOPSONS, in High-Street.
MDCCLXXI.

LEWER, Sidney H., b.1862
398 British poultry and poultry keeping / by Sidney H. Lewer; with an introduction by Edward Brown. — 3rd ed. — London: Produced and published for the Congress Committee for Great Britain by "The Feathered World", [1927]. — 116p, [31]p of plates: ill (some col.); 25cm

LEWIS, William M.
399 The people's practical poultry book: a work on the breeds, breeding, rearing and general management of poultry / by Wm. M. Lewis. — New York: American News Co., 1871. — 223p: ill; 24cm

LIBERATI, Francesco
400 La perfettione del cavallo, libri tre / di Francesco Liberati Romano ...; et insieme dell'arte di caualcare di Senofonte, tradotto dal greco nel nostro idioma italiano. — In Roma: Per gli heredi di Francesco Corbelletti, 1639. — [8], 56, 9-24, 73-82, [2] (blank), 33-183p: ill; 21cm (4to)

LIGHTBODY, James
401 Every man his own gauger: wherein not only the artist is shown a more ready and exact method of gauging ... / by J. Lightbody philomath. — London: Printed for G.C. ..., [17--?]. — [4], 68p; 15cm (12mo)
Bound with: The compleat husbandman / by G. Markham.— London: G. Conyers, 1707

LINCOLNSHIRE GRAZIER
see HORNE, T. H. (Thomas Hartwell), 1780-1862

402 **LIST OF SHEEP MARKS**: for the counties of Aberdeen, Banff, Kincardine, Forfar, and part of Perthshire – Glenshee / compiled by a committee of sheep farmers. — Aberdeen: Printed at the Free Press Office, 1878. — 88p; 18cm

403 **LIST OF SHEEP MARKS**: for the counties of Aberdeen, Banff, Forfar, Kincardine, Elgin and Moray, Nairn, and Inverness / compiled by a committee of sheep farmers. — Aberdeen: Printed at the "Free Press" Office, 1897. — [4], 224p; 20cm

LITTLE, John
404 Practical observations on the improvement and management of mountain sheep, and sheep farms: also, remarks on stock of various kinds / by John Little. — Second edition. — Edinburgh: Printed by John Moir ... for Macredie, Skelly, and Muckersy, Edinburgh; and Longman, Hurst, Rees, Orme & Brown, London, 1818. — [4], iii, [1] (blank), iv, [9]-198p; 23cm (8vo)
Colophon reads: Printed by John Moir, Edinburgh, 1815
Chapter VII consists of Observations on the improvement of the country by means of rail-ways

LIVINGSTON, Robert R., 1746-1813

405 Essay on sheep: their varieties – account of the merinoes of Spain, France, &c. ... / by Robert R. Livingston ... — New York: Printed by T. and J. Swords ..., 1809. — 186p; 21cm (8vo)
Pages [3]-4 are bound at the end

LONG, James

406 Poultry for prizes and profit: being practical details for the breeding, management and exhibition of domestic fowls / by James Long. — London: L. Upcott Gill, [1890?]. — iv, 204p, [26] leaves of plates: ill; 20cm
Pages 82*-85* inserted between p.88-89

LOWSON, G. (George)

407 The complete cattle doctor: comprising the causes, symptoms, and most approved methods, for the prevention and cure of the various diseases of cows, oxen, sheep, and swine ... / by G. Lowson. — 9th ed. — London: Jones & Co., [184-?]. — [3]-352p: ill; 13cm (8vo)

408 The modern farrier: a treatise on the causes, symptoms, and most approved methods of preventing and curing the various diseases of horses, cows, calves, sheep, and hogs / by G. Lowson; corrected and improved by Robert Armstrong. — 99th ed. — Otley: W. Walker and Sons, [18--]. — 224p: ill; 18cm (8vo)

409 The modern farrier: containing the causes, symptoms, and most approved methods of preventing and curing the various diseases of horses, cows, oxen, sheep, swine, and dogs ... / by G. Lowson. — London: Published by Jones and Co. ..., [1836?]. — [4], x, [5]-608p, [8] leaves of plates: ill; 22cm (4to)
Date on spine: 1830

410 The modern farrier: containing the causes, symptoms, and most approved methods of preventing and curing the various diseases of horses and dogs ... / by George Lowson. — 10th ed. — London: Jones & Co., 1841. — 384p: ill; 13cm (8vo)

411 The modern farrier: containing the causes, symptoms, and most approved methods of preventing and curing the various diseases of horses, cows, and sheep ... / by G. Lowson. — London: H.G. Collins, 1851. — 192p: ill; 18cm
Ms note inserted

412 Lowson's Modern farrier: a treatise on the causes, symptoms, and most approved methods of preventing & curing the various diseases of horses, cows, calves, sheep and hogs / corrected and improved by Robert Armstrong. — London: W. Walker and Sons, [1877?]. — 255p: ill; 16cm
The first and last leaves are used as paste-down endpapers in the publisher's binding of decorative colour printed paper covered boards

LUND, James
413 The new cattle doctor: comprising the nature of the diseases to which cattle, sheep, and swine are liable ... / by James Lund. — Wakefield: W. Nicholson and Sons, [18--]. — 381, [1]p: col.ill; 13cm (8vo)
At head of title: The farmers friend

M., F.
The jockey's guide
see F.M.

M.S.
414 The country-man's jewel: or, The jockey's master-piece ... / by M.S. gent. L.M. J. Lambert, and others. — London: Printed for G. Conyers ..., [17--]. — 118p; 15cm (12mo)
Preface signed: L.M., J.L., A.S.
Alternative title on A2 (verso): The husbandman, farmer, and grazier's compleat instructor, in feeding, brooding, buying, and selling cattle
Imperfect: 1st and last leaf missing (A1, G8)

415 The country-man's jewel: or, The jockey's master-piece ... / by M.S. gent. L.M. J. Lambert, and others. — Glasgow: Printed by John Hall ..., 1750. — 118, [2]p: ill; 15cm (12mo)
Preface signed: L.M., J.L., A.S.
This work appears to have three alternative title pages, the first two leaves consisting of:
A1 (recto): coarse wood-cuts of a bull, cow, and pig in compartments. See note under A.S. (4)
A1 (verso): The country-mam's [sic] treasure: shewing the nature, causes, and cure of all diseases incident to cattle ... by A.S. and improv'd by J. Lambert
A2 (recto): (the title given above)
A2 (verso): The husbandman, farmer, and grazier's compleat instructor, in feeding, brooding, buying, and selling cattle

MACKENZIE, Sir George Steuart, 1780-1848
416 A treatise on the diseases and management of sheep: with introductory remarks on their anatomical structure ... / by Sir George Steuart Mackenzie, bart. — Edinburgh; [London]: Printed for Archibald Constable & Co. Edinburgh; Constable, Hunter, Park & Hunter, and John Harding, London; by J. Young, Inverness, 1809. — viii, [9]-180p, V leaves of plates: ill; 23cm (8vo)

MAIN, James, 1775?-1846
417 A treatise on the breeding, rearing and fattening of poultry / by James Main. — 3rd ed. — London: Ridgways, 1839. — 340, [2]p; 20cm (12mo)

418 A treatise on the breeding, rearing and fattening of poultry / by James Main. — 4th ed. — London: James Ridgway, 1847. — 340, [2]p; 20cm (12mo)

MAPLES, John

419 The new complete horse doctor: or, horseman's sure guide: and every man his own farrier ... / by John Maples ... — London: Printed for Alex. Hogg, [178-]. — iii, [4]-8, [13]-212 [i.e.112]p., [1] leaf of plates: ill; 18cm (12mo)
Page 112 misnumbered as 212

MARKHAM, Gervase, 1568?-1637

420 Cavelarice, or The English horseman: contayning all the arte of horse-manship ... / by Geruase Markham. — [London: Printed for Edward White ..., 1607]. — [16], 88, [4], 264, [4], 72, [4], 54, [4], 56, [4], 64, [4], 81, [1] (blank), [4], 40p: ill; 19cm (4to)
Each pt. has special t.p.
Imprint from t.p. of "the second booke"
Lacks plate
The works of Gervase Markham are comprehensively described in Poynter, F.N.L., A bibliography of Gervase Markham, 1568?-1637 (804)

421 Cavalarice, or The English horseman: contayning all the art of horse-manship ... / by Geruase Markham. — Newly imprinted, corrected & augmented ... — [London: Printed by Edw. Allde for Edward White], 1617. — [16], 88, [4], 264, [4], 84, [4], 57, [1] (blank), [4], 58, [4], 67, [1] (blank), [4], 86, [4], 37p: ill; 19cm (4to)
Books 2-8 have special title pages, 4-8 are dated 1617
Imprint partly from t.p. of book 2

422 [Cheape and good husbandry. Selections] The compleat horseman / by Gervase Markham; ... edited by Dan Lucid; with pictures by Pauline Baynes. — London: Robson Books, 1976. — 76, [3]p: ill; 25cm
Ill. on lining papers
'... adapted from "Cheape and good husbandry", published by Gervase Markham in 1614' — title page verso

423 The citizen and countryman's experienced farrier ... / by J. Markham, G. Jefferies, and experienced Indians. — Chambersburg: Printed by Thomas J. Wright, 1839. — 332, [9]p; 18cm (12mo)

424 The compleat husbandman and gentleman's recreation: or, the whole art of husbandry ... / by G. Markham gent. — London: Printed for G. Conyers ..., 1707. — [4], 38p: ill; 15cm (12mo)
See notes re text, and re the frontispiece plate, under A.S. (2,4)
Bound with: The husbandman's jewel. — London: Conyers, [1720?]; Every man his own gauger / by J. Lightbody. — London: G.C., [17--?] and A new book of knowledge. — London: Conyers, 1697

425 The compleat jockey: or the most exact rules and methods ... / attributed to Gervase Markham gentleman. — London: Woodstock, 1933. — 93p; 23cm
Copy no. 479 of a limited edition of 500

426 The country gentleman's companion: in two volumes ... / by a country gentleman, from his own experience. — London: Printed for the author, and sold by T. Trye ..., 1753. — 2v.in 1 ([8], [13]-239; [4], 172, [64]p); 18cm (12mo)
Vol. 2 has separate t.p. and half title
Attributed to G. Markham. Cf. Poynter, 35

427 The English husbandman: the first part: contayning the knowledge of the true nature of euery soyle within this kingdome ... / by G. M. — London: Printed by T.S. for Iohn Browne ..., 1613. — [76], 132p: ill, plans; 19cm (4to)
Imperfect: some leaves mutilated with loss of text. Bound with: The second booke of the English husbandman / by G.M. — London: T.S. for I. Browne, 1615

428 The second booke of the English husbandman: contayning the ordering of the kitchin-garden ... / by G. M. — London: Printed by T.S. for Iohn Browne ..., 1615. — [2] (blank), [14], 205 [i.e. 105]p; 19cm (4to)
Without The pleasures of princes. Bound with: The English husbandman / by G.M. — London: T.S. for I. Browne, 1613

429 The English husbandman: drawne into two bookes ... — Newlie reviewed, corrected, and inlarged / by the first author, G.M. — London: Printed for William Sheares ..., 1635. — [14], 227, [15], 96, [2], 54p: ill; 20cm (4to)
The seconde booke and The pleasures of princes have special title pages and separate pagination

430 The gentleman's accomplish'd jockey: with the compleat horseman, and approved farrier ... / by G. M. gent. — London: Printed for H. Tracy ..., 1722. — 156, [12]p, [1] folded leaf of plates: ill; 15cm (12mo)

431 Hungers preuention: or, The whole arte of fowling: by water and land ... / by Gervase Markham. — London: Printed by A. Math. for Anne Helme and Thomas Langley ..., 1621. — [14], 285p: ill; 15cm (8vo)
Imperfect: frontispiece missing, t.p. mutilated, restored with loss of imprint date

432 Hungers prevention: or, The whole art of fowling: by water and land ... / by Gervase Markham. — London: Printed for Francis Grove, and are to be sold by Martha Harrison ..., 1655. — [16], 285p: ill; 14cm (8vo)

433 Markhams faithfull farrier: wherein the depth of his skill is laid open ... — London: Printed by G. P. for Tho. Vere ..., 1667. — [14], 110, [2]p: ill; 15cm (8vo)
Imperfect: A1, E2 and H2 missing

434 Markhams maister-peece. Or, what doth a horse-man lacke: containing all possible knowledge ... / written by Geruase Markham gentleman. — London: Printed by Nicholas Okes, and are to be sold by Arthur Iohnson ..., 1610. — [8], 506, [4]p, [1] folded leaf of plates: ill; 18cm (4to)
Some ms notes
Illustrations: page 108 and 109

MARKHAMS
MAISTER-PEECE.
OR,
What doth a Horse-man lacke.

Containing all possible knowledge whatsoeuer which doth belong to any Smith, Farrier or Horse-leech, *touching the curing of all maner of diseases or sorrances* in horses; drawne with great paine and most approued *experience from the publique practise of all the forraine Horse-*Marshals of Christendome, and from the priuate practise of all *the best Farriers of this kingdome.*

Being deuided into two Bookes.

The first containing all cures Physicall. The Second whatsoeuer belongeth to Chirurgerie, with *an addition of* 130 *most principall Chapters,* and 340 *most* excellent medicines, receits and secrets worthy euery mans knowledge, *neuer written of, nor mentioned in* any Author before whatsoeuer.

Together with the true nature, vse, and qualitie of *euerie Simple spoken of through the whole worke.*

Reade me, practise me, and admire me.

Written by *Geruase Markham* Gentleman.

Pro. 12. ver. 10.
A iust man hath pity on his beast: but the mercies of the wicked are cruell.

LONDON,
Printed by *Nicholas Okes,* and are to be sold by *Arthur Iohnson,* dwelling at the signe of the white horse, neere the great North doore of S. *Pauls* Church. 1610.

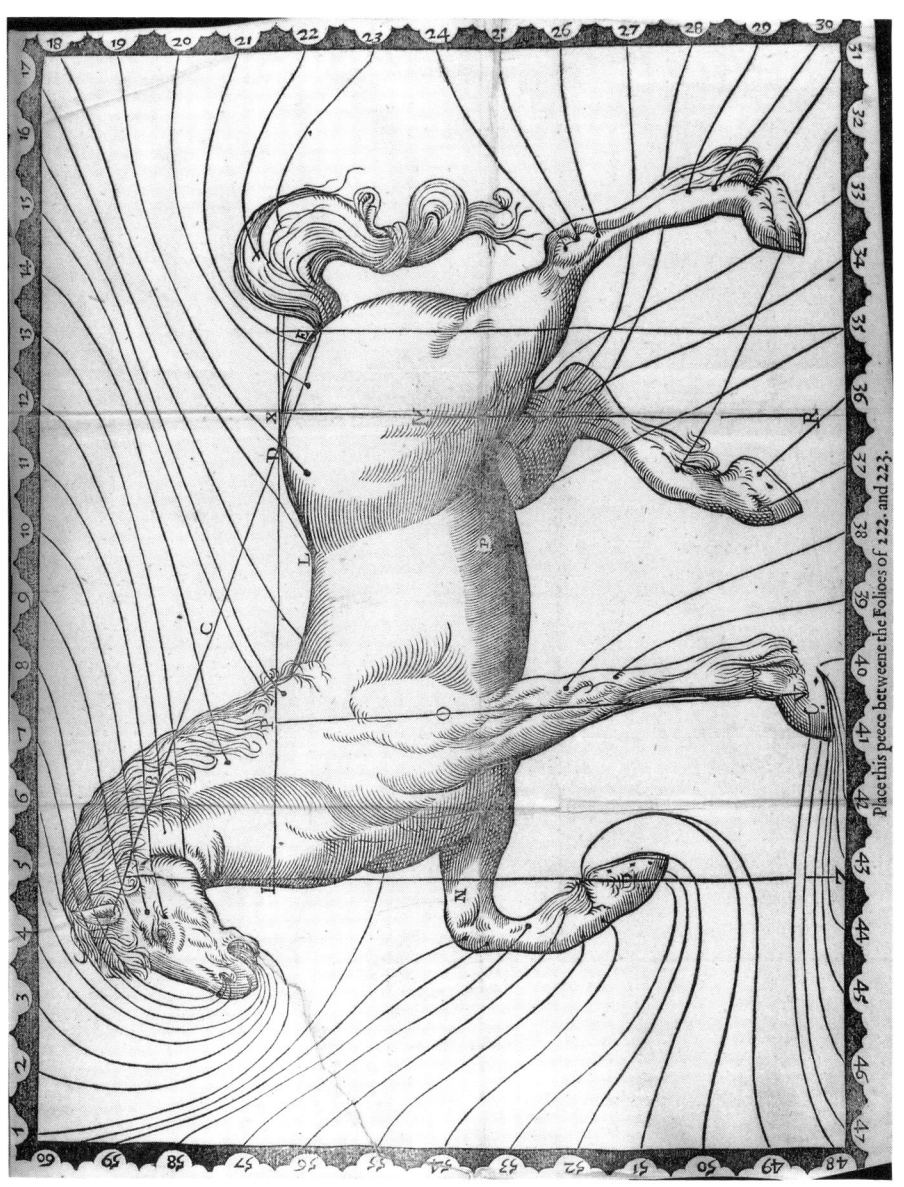

Markham 1610 (434)

435 Markhams maister-peece: containing all knowledge belonging to a smith, farrier, or horse-leach ... being diuided into two bookes ... / writtten [sic] by Gervase Markham. — Now newly imprinted, corrected and augmented ... — Imprinted at London: By Nicholas Okes, 1615. — [16], 565p: ill; 19cm (4to)
Additional engraved t.p. with: "The second impression". The second booke has special t.p.
Spine lettered: Markham's Horse cures
Lacks the large folded plate, the stub of which is present between p.242 and 243
Bookplate of Algernon Capell, Earl of Essex ... 1701, on verso of A2

436 Markhams maister-peece: contayning all knowledge belonging to the smith, farrier, or horse-leech ... being diuided into two bookes ... / written by Gervase Markham, gent. — Now the fourth time newly imprinted, corrected, and augmented ... — Imprinted at London: By Nicholas Okes and are to be sold by Nicholas Fussell and Humphrey Mosley ..., 1631. — [12], 587, [8]p: ill; 19cm (4to)
Additional engraved t.p. The second booke has special t.p. dated 1630
Lacks the folded plate

437 Markhams maister-peece: contayning all knowledge belonging to the smith, farrier, or horse-leech ... being divided into two bookes ... / written by Gervase Markham, gent. — Now the sixt time newly imprinted, corrected, and augmented ... — Imprinted at London: By John Okes ..., 1643. — [15], 591, [22]p, [1] folded leaf of plates: ill; 19cm (4to)
Additional engraved t.p. dated 1644. The second booke has special t.p.

438 Markhams maister-peece: containing all knowledge belonging to the smith, farrier, or horse-leech ... / written by Gervase Markham, gent. — Now the eighth time newly imprinted, corrected, and augmented ... — Imprinted at London: By W. Wilson, and are to be sold by George Sawbridge ..., 1656. — [15], 591, [22]p, [1] folded leaf of plates: ill; 19cm (4to)
Additional engraved t.p.

439 Markham's master-piece revived: containing all knowledge belonging to the smith, farrier, or horse-leach, touching the curing all diseases, in horses ... — Now the fourteenth time printed, corrected and augmented ... — London: Printed by John Richardson for Tho. Passinger ... and M. Wotton and George Coniers ..., 1688. — [15], 394, [2], 26, 49, [3]p, [1] folded leaf of plates: ill; 20cm (4to)
Additional engraved t.p. with: "The 11th impression"

440 Markham's master-piece: containing all knowledge belonging to the smith, farrier, or horse-leach ... also The compleat jockey ... — London: Printed for A. Bettesworth ... [and 5 others], 1734. — [8], 318, iii, 2-64p: ill; 23cm (4to)
Additional engraved t.p. with: "The 21st impression"

441 Markham's method or epitome: wherein is shewed his approved remedies ... / by Gervase Markham, gentleman. — The eleventh edition / corrected by the author. — London: Printed for William Thackeray ..., 1684. — [10], 86p: ill; 15cm (8vo)
Additional engraved t.p.
Bound with: The secrets of Albertus Magnus. — London: M.H. and T.M., [1691?]

442 The perfect horseman: or the experienced secrets of Mr. Markham's fifty years practice: shewing how a man may come to be a general horseman ... / and now published by Lancelot Thetford ... — London: Printed for Humphrey Moseley ..., 1656. — [14], 175p, [1] leaf of plates: ill; 15cm (8vo)
20p advertisement of H. Moseley bound in
Illustration: page 112

443 The perfect horse-man or the experienced secrets of Mr. Markhams fifty years practise: shewing how a man may come to be a general horseman ... / and now published by Lancelot Thetford ... — London: Printed for Humphrey Moseley ..., 1660[?]. — [14], 175p, [1] leaf of plates: ill; 15cm (8vo)
Imperfect: t.p. mutilated with loss of text. Cropped copy

444 A way to get wealth: containing six principal vocations, or callings ... / the first five books gathered by G.M. The last by Master W.L. for the benefit of Great Brittain. — The thirteenth time corrected, and augmented / by the author. — London: Printed by E.H. for George Sawbridge ..., 1676. — 6v.in 1: ill; 20cm (4to)
Each book has special t.p. and separate pagination
Contents: Cheap and good husbandry, for the well-ordering of all beasts and fowls. 13th ed. 1676 — Country contentments. Or, The husbandmans recreations. 11th ed. 1675 — The English house-wife. 1675 — The inrichment of the Weald of Kent. 1675 — Markham's farewel to husbandry: or, The enriching of all sorts of barren and sterile grounds. 1676 — A new orchard & garden ... With The country house-wifes garden ... by William Lawson. 1676

MARTIN, W. C. L. (William Charles Linnaeus), 1798-1864
445 Our domestic fowls and song birds / by W.C.L. Martin. — London: The Religious Tract Society, [1847?]. — [2], 192, 192p, [1] leaf of plates: ill; 15cm (16mo)

MASCALL, Leonard, d.1589
446 The first [-third] booke of cattel: wherein is shewed, the gouernement of oxen, kine, and calues ... / gathered and set foorth by Leonard Mascall. — At Lodon [sic]: Printed by Iohn Harison ..., 1600. — [6], 301, [1]p: ill; 19cm (4to)
Each book has separate t.p. and index
Reference: STC 17583

447 The first [-third] booke of cattell: wherein is shewed, the gouernement of oxen, kine, and calues ... / gathered and set forth by Leonard Mascall. — At London: Printed by Iohn Harison ..., 1605. — [8], 301, [1]p; 19cm (4to)
Many errors in pagination. Each book has separate t.p. and index
Reference: STC 17584

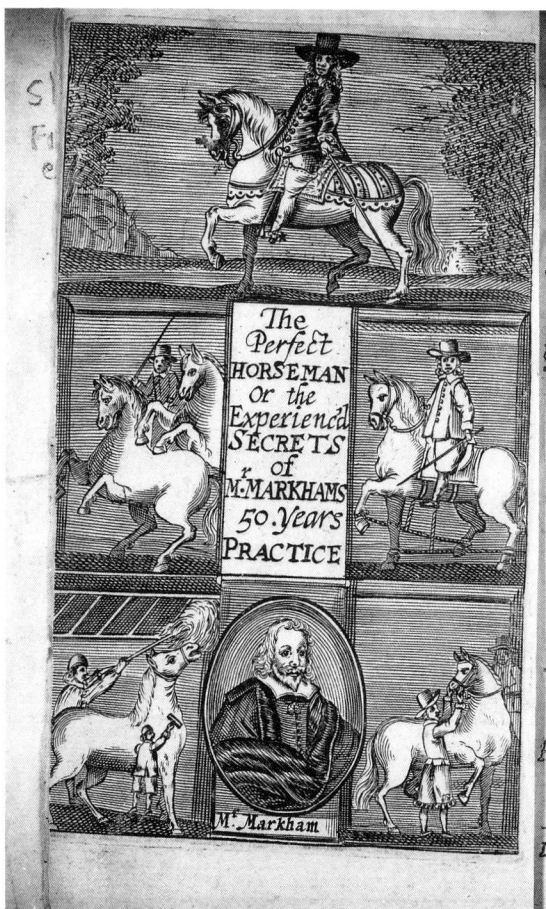

THE PERFECT HORSEMAN:

OR THE Experienced Secrets

OF

Mr. MARKHAM'S Fifty Years Practice.

Shewing how a man may come to be a General Horseman, By the knowledge of these Seven Offices; VIZ.

The { Breeder, Rider, Feeder, Keeper, Ambler, Buyer, } FARRYER.

Never Printed before.

And now Published by *Lancelot Thetford*, Practitioner in the same Art for the space of Forty Years.

LONDON, Printed for *Humphrey Moseley*, at the Prince's Arms in St. *Pauls* Church-yard. 1656.

448 The gouernment of cattell: diuided into three books ... / gathered by Leonard Mascal. — London: Printed by Thomas Harper for Iohn Harison ..., 1633. — [6], 307, [2]p; 19cm (4to)
Each book has separate t.p. and index
Reference: STC 17588

449 The government of cattell: divided into three books ... / gathered by Leonard Mascal. — London: Printed by Thomas Harper, for Martha Harison ..., 1653. — [6], 308, [1]p; 19cm (4to)
Each book has separate t.p. and index. Imprint of 2nd and 3rd book is: London: Printed by E. Alsop for Martha Harrison ..., 1653
Reference: Wing (2nd ed.) M902

450 The government of cattel: divided into three books ... / gathered by Leonard Mascal. — London: Printed for William Gilbertson, and John Stafford ..., 1662. — [6], 307, [2]p; 18cm (4to)
Each book has separate t.p. and index. Date of imprint of books 2 & 3 is 1661
Reference: Wing (2nd ed.) M903
Some ms. notes

451 The countreyman's jewel: or, the government of cattel: divided into three books ... / gathered at first by Leonard Mascal, but much inlarged by Rich. Ruscam, gent. — London: Printed for William Thackery ..., 1680. — [16], 383, [33]p, [3] leaves of plates (2 folded): ill; 17cm (8vo)
Each book has separate t.p. and index. Additional engraved t.p.
Reference: Wing (2nd ed.) M898

452 The husbandlye ordring and gouernmente of poultrie: practised by the learnedste, and suche as haue bene knowne skilfullest in that arte, and in our tyme. — Imprinted at London: By Thomas Purfoote, for Gerarde Dewse, 1581 ([19--] photocopy). — 1v.; 19cm
By Leonard Mascall
A facsimile made from the BL copy. No other edition is recorded

MAYHEW, Edward, 1813?-1868
453 The horse's mouth, showing the age by the teeth: containing a full description of the periods when the teeth are cut ... / by Edward Mayhew. — 2nd ed. — London: Messrs. Fores, [18--]. — xii, 194p, [9] leaves of col. plates: ill; 23cm
First ed. published: 1849

MÉGNIN, Paul, b.1868
454 Le livre d'or de la santé des animaux domestiques: mémento pratique de zootechnie et d'hygiène ... / par Paul Mégnin; préface de M.P. Dechambre. — Paris: Bong & Cie, [1905]. — x, 56, [34]p, [17] leaves of plates: ill (some col.), multi-layered models; 30cm
Paul-Henri Mégnin was the son of Jean-Pierre Mégnin, military veterinary surgeon and prolific author and artist

MERINO SOCIETY

455 Report of the Merino Society: established 4th March, 1811 ... — Nottingham; London: The Society, 1811-1813. — 21cm (4to)
Holdings: 1st — 3rd
Receipt for life subscription of J. Tharp laid in

MERRICK, William

456 The classical farrier: exhibiting the whole anatomy of that noble animal the horse ... / by William Merrick, farrier, assisted by several eminent physicians, anatomists, and professors of surgery. — London: Printed by J. Aspin ... and sold by J. and W. Stratford ..., 1788. — [10], xxiv, 25-827p, VII leaves of plates: ill; 22cm (8vo)

MILES, W. J. (William J.)

457 Modern practical farriery: a complete system of the veterinary art as at present practised at the Royal Veterinary College, London / by W.J. Miles; including practical treatises on Cattle ... by John Walker ... — London: William Mackenzie, 1868-1869. — 16pts: col.ill; 32cm
Copy 1: In parts as issued
Copy 2: Bound vol. published 1899? ([2], 180, vii, 181-538, vi, 96p., [48] leaves of plates: col.ill; 31cm)
Miles' Modern practical farriery was issued variously in 16 monthly parts; in 5 quarterly parts; and in a number of editions as a single quarto volume. It consists of four sections: Varieties and management of the horse; A compendium of veterinary knowledge (Division II); Cattle: their management in dairy, field, and stall (Division III); and, The diseases and treatment of cattle, sheep, and pigs. Numbers and states of plates were varied between editions, and both the distribution of the plates throughout the volume, and the order of binding the four sections and the Index etc appear to have been left to the discretion of individual binders. Thus different plates have been chosen to be used as a frontispiece in individual copies

MILES, William

458 The horse's foot: and how to keep it sound / by William Miles. — 5th ed. with an appendix. — London: Longman, Brown, Green, and Longman, 1847. — x, 59, 31, [21]p, 10 leaves of plates: ill; 28cm (4to)
Presented to Lady Rolle by the author (inscription)

MILLS, John, d.1784

459 The modern system of farriery: showing the most approved methods of breeding, rearing, and fitting for use, all kinds of horses ... / by John Mills, esq. ... — Boston: Printed and sold by William Spotswood, 1796. — [4], 274, [10]p; 17cm (12mo)

460 A treatise on cattle: shewing the most approved methods of breeding, rearing, and fitting for use, horses, asses, ... / carefully collected from the best authorities, and interspersed with remarks, by John Mills, esq. ... — Dublin: Printed for W. Whitestone ... [and 8 others], 1776. — viii, 456, [16]p; 21cm (8vo)
Erratum: on last p.

MONTAGUE, Peregrine

461 The family pocket-book: or, fountain of true and useful knowledge: containing the farrier's guide ... / compiled after thirty years experience, by Peregrine Montague, gent. — London: Printed for George Paul ..., [1796?]. — 166p: ill; 18cm (12mo)
The gardener's legacy / by Charles Knight: p.100-125. — The good housewife's daily companion / taken chiefly from the late Sir Hans Sloane, and the ingenious Dr. Lower's works: p.[126]-159
Four cuttings pasted onto the endpapers

MOORCROFT, William, 1765?-1825

462 Cursory account of the various methods of shoeing horses, hitherto practised: with incidental observations / by William Moorcroft. — London: Printed by W. Bulmer and Co. ... and sold by G. and W. Nicol ... Wright ... and Sewell ..., 1800. — xi, [1] (blank), 60p: ill; 20cm (8vo)
Errata slip pasted on last p.

463 Travels in the Himalayan provinces of Hindustan and the Panjab: in Ladakh and Kashmir; in Peshawar, Kabul, Kunduz, and Bokhara / by William Moorcroft and George Trebeck; prepared for the press from original journals and correspondence by Horace Hayman Wilson. — London: John Murray, 1841. — 2v (lvi, 459p, [2] leaves of plates (1 folded); viii, 508p, [1] leaf of plates): ill, map; 22cm (8vo)
Provenance: J.W. Barber-Lomax

MORE, Sir J. (Jonas), 1617-1679

464 Englands interest: or, the gentleman and farmers friend: shewing, 1. How land may be improv'd from 20s to 8l. and so to 100l per acre, per annum ... / by Sir J. More. — The fourth edition. — London: Printed and sold by J. How ..., 1707. — [2], 166, [1]p; 15cm (12mo)
Reference: Rothamsted cat. (1926), p.94

MORGAN, George
The new complete sportsman
see FAIRFAX, Thomas

MORGAN, Nicholas

465 The perfection of horse-manship: drawne from nature; arte, and practise / by Nicholas Morgan of Crolane, in the countye of Kent, gent. — Imprinted at London: For Edward White, and are to be solde at his shop ..., 1609. — [28], 272, [4], 273-145 [i.e. 345], [4]p: ill; 19cm (4to)
Errata: last p.
Errors in pagination: p.344-345 misnumbered as 144-145
Illustration: page 116

Vp and be doing, and the Lord will be with thee.
1. *Chron.* 22. 16.

THE
PERFECTION
of HORSE-MANSHIP,
drawne from Nature; Arte,
and Practise.

By *Nicholas Morgan* of *Crolane*, in
the Countye of *Kent*, Gent.

Data fata sequutus.

Τῷ πρωτοπείρῳ συγγνώμη.

Nil tam facile, quam otiosum et dormientem de aliorum labore, et vigilijs disputare. Hier.

ῥᾷον μωμεῖσθαι ἢ μιμεῖσθαι.

Imprinted at London for *Edward VVhite*, and
are to be solde at his shop at the Signe of the
Gun, neere the little North dore of Saint
Paules. 1609.

466 The horse-mans honour: or, The beautie of horse-manship: as the choice, natures, breeding, breaking, riding, and dieting, whether outlandish or English horses ... — London: Printed for Iohn Marriott ..., 1620. — [14], 144[i.e.344]p; 19cm (4to)
Reissue of: The perfection of horse-manship, by Nicholas Morgan, 1609
Reference: STC (2nd ed.) 18105.3
Imperfect: A1 (blank), A4, Y1 and Y8 missing. Bound with: Browne his fiftie yeares practice / by William Browne. — [London]: Nicholas Okes, 1624
Not recognised by Smith, who, although he had not seen a copy, attributed the work to Markham (Smith, I, 278)
Illustration: page 118

MORRELL, L. A. (Luke A.)
467 The American shepherd: being a history of the sheep, with their breeds, management, and diseases ... / by L.A. Morrell. — New York: Harper & Brothers, 1863. — xxii, [13]-437p: ill; 20cm

MORTIMER, J. (John), 1656?-1736
468 The whole art of husbandry; or, the way of managing and improving of land: being a full collection of what hath been writ ... / by J. Mortimer, esq. ... — The second edition, corrected. — London: Printed by J.H. for H. Mortlock ... and J. Robinson ..., 1708. — [16], 632, [8]p: ill; 20cm (8vo)
Errata: on last p.

MORTON, W. J. T. (William John Thomas), 1800-1868
469 A manual of pharmacy: for the student of veterinary medicine ... / by W.J.T. Morton. — London: Longman and Co., [1837]. — vii, 188p, [1] folded leaf of plates; 18cm (8vo)

470 On calculous concretions in the horse, ox, sheep, and dog: being the substance of two essays read before the Veterinary Medical Association / by W.J.T. Morton. — London: Longman, Brown, Green & Longmans, 1844. — [2], iv, [2], 94p, IV leaves of plates: col.ill; 23cm (4to)

MOUBRAY, Bonington
see LAWRENCE, John, 1753-1839

MURRELL, James
471 Valuable recipes: for neat stock, horses, sheep, pigs, and dogs; and some others, which will be found equally serviceable to the human frame, and for domestic purposes / collected, and made use of for more than thirty years, by James Murrell ... — [Little Cressingham]: Printed for the author, by Gedge and Barker, Bury, 1823. — 77p; 23cm (8vo)
Not known to Smith. Not in RVC or RCVS

The Horse-mans Honour:
Or, The
BEAVTIE
OF HORSE-
MANSHIP.

AS

The Choise, Natures, Breeding, Break-
ing, Riding, and Dieting, whether Outlandish or English Horses.

With the true, easie, Cheape, and most Approued
manner, how to know and Cure all Diseases
in any Horse whatsoeuer.

Not innented and drawne from Forraigne Nations,
but by long Experience and Knowledge of many
yeares Practise: And now published at the request
of diuers Honorable and worthy Persons,
for the generall good of this noble
Nation of *Great Britaine*.

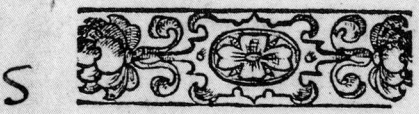

LONDON,
Printed for *Iohn Marriott*, and are to be sould at his Shop in St.
Dunstons Churchyard in Fleetstreet. 1620.

N.B.
472 The farrier's and horseman's dictionary: being a compleat system of horsemanship ... / by N.B. Philippos. — London: Printed for J. Darby [and 8 others], 1726. — viii, 454, [1]p; 21cm (8vo)
Philippos transliterated from the Greek
Printed in columns

NAISMITH, John
473 Observations on the different breeds of sheep and the state of sheep farming: in the southern districts of Scotland: being the result of a tour through these parts, made under the direction of The Society for Improvement of British Wool / by John Naismyth at Hamilton. — Edinburgh: Printed by W. Smellie ..., 1795. — [2], 75p; 25cm (4to)
Disbound. Imperfect: first leaf missing

NAPIER, William John, 1786-1834
474 A treatise on practical store-farming: as applicable to the mountainous region of Etterick Forest, and the pastoral district of Scotland in general / by the Honourable William John Napier. — Edinburgh: Waugh and Innes, 1822. — [iii]-viii, 280p, [3] leaves of plates (2 folded): ill, map; 22cm (8vo)

475 The **NEW AND COMPLETE UNIVERSAL VERMIN-KILLER**: being an infallible directory ... — London: Jones and Co., 1824. — 59p, [1] folded leaf of plates: ill; 18cm (12mo)
Bound with: The complete dog fancier. — London: T. Hughes, 1824; The complete pigeon & rabbit fancier. — London: T. Hughes, 1824; The domestic poultry instructor. — London: T. Hughes, [1824?] and The British bird fancier. — London: T. Hughes, 1824

476 A **NEW BOOK OF KNOWLEDGE**: treating of things, whereof some are profitable, some precious, and some pleasant and delightful ... — London: Printed for G. Con[y]ers ..., 1697. — 12p; 15cm (12mo)
Bound with: The compleat husbandman / by G. Markham. — London: G. Conyers, 1707

NEWCASTLE, William Cavendish, Duke of, 1592-1676
477 A new method, and extraordinary invention to dress horses: and work them according to nature ... / by the thrice noble, high, and puissant Prince William Cavendishe ... — London: Printed by Tho. Milbourn, 1667. — [12], 342, 8, 343-352, [4]p; 36cm (fol.)

478 A general system of horsemanship: in all it's branches ... Vol.II. — London: Printed for C. Corbett ... and sold by J. Joliffe ..., 1748. — [2], [6], 4, [2], 5-36, 33-138, [14]p, [20] leaves of plates (some folded): ill; 45cm (fol.)
Vol.1 is a translation of Méthode et invention nouvelle de dresser les chevaux by William Cavendish, duke of Newcastle, originally published: Antwerp, 1657; v.2 is translation of La parfaite connoissance des chevaux by Jean de Saunier
Edited by John Brindley
Reference: Brunet, v.1, col.1700

OPERA DELLA MEDICINA DE CAVALLI
see HIPPIATRICA

OSMER, William
479 A dissertation on horses: wherein it is demonstrated ... that innate qualities do not exist ... / by William Osmer. — London: Printed for T. Waller ..., 1756. — [2], 61, [3]p; 21cm (8vo)
Bound with: Observations and discoveries made upon horses / by the Sieur La Fosse. — London: J. Nourse, 1755

480 A treatise on the diseases and lameness of horses / by W. Osmer. — London: Printed for T. Waller ..., 1759. — [2], 125, [1]p; 18cm (8vo)
Two copies

481 A treatise on the diseases and lameness of horses: in which is laid down a proper method of shoeing ... / by W. Osmer. — London: Printed for T. Waller ... and A. Chapelle ..., 1761. — [2], 2, 300, [1]p; 21cm (8vo)
Errata: on p.300

PALMIERI, Lorenzino
482 Perfette regole, et modi di cavalcare / di Lorenzino Palmieri fiorentino ... — In Venetia: Appresso Barezzo Barezzi. Ad istanza di Paolo Frambotto libraro in Padoua, 1625. — [8], 112, [1] folded leaf of plates: ill; 23cm (4to)
Added engraved t.p. dated 1626

PARKES, Samuel, 1759-1825
483 A letter to the farmers and graziers of Great Britain, on the advantages of using salt in the various branches of agriculture, and in feeding all kinds of farming stock / by Samuel Parkes ... — The third edition, corrected. — London: Published by Baldwin, Cradock, and Joy ... and sold by J.M. Richardson ... [and 4 others], 1819. — xi, [12]-106, [1]p; 22cm (8vo)

484 **PARKINSON,** Richard, 1748-1815
Treatise on the breeding and management of livestock: comprising cattle, sheep ... / by Richard Parkinson ... — London: Printed for Cadell and Davies ... and R. Scholey ..., 1810. — 2v ([8], xxxii, 436p, [3] leaves of plates;[8], 484, [16]p, [5] leaves of plates): ill; 22cm (8vo)

PARKINSON, Thomas
485 A treatise on the management of parturient animals: in two parts / by T. Parkinson ... — Nottingham: Printed and sold by H. Barnett ..., 1812. — xii, 118p; 21cm
Imperfect: plate missing

PARRY, Caleb Hillier, 1755-1822

486 Communications to the Board of Agriculture: on subjects relative to the husbandry, and internal improvement of the country. Vol.V, part II, no.XVIII: An essay on the nature, produce, origin, and extension of the Merino breed of sheep: to which is added a history of a cross of that breed with Ryeland ewes ... / by Caleb Hilliar [sic] Parry ... — London: Printed by W. Bulmer and Co. for G. and W. Nicol ... and to the Board of Agriculture; sold by Wilkie and Robinson ... [and 4 others], 1807. — viii, [337]-541, [17]p; 30cm (4to)
Errata: on last p.

487 Facts and observations tending to shew the practicability and advantage to the individual and the nation, of producing in the British Isles clothing wool: equal to that of Spain ... / by Caleb Hillier Parry ... — Bath: Printed by R. Cruttwell; [London]: and sold by Cadell and Davies ..., 1800. — [4], 93, [3]p; 25cm (4to)
Corrigenda: last p.

PEALL, Thomas

488 A treatise on the foot-rot in sheep: including remarks on the exciting cause, method of cure ... being the substance of three lectures delivered in the theatre of the Royal Dublin Society / by Thomas Peall. — Dublin: Printed by Joshua Porter, 1822. — ix, 55p; 21cm (4to)

PEARSON, Leonard, 1868-1909

489 Diseases of poultry / by Leonard Pearson. Enemies of poultry; by B.H. Warren. — [Harrisburg, Pa.]: Clarence M. Busch, 1897. — 116, xxiv, 750p, [105] leaves of plates (1 folded): ill (some col.); 25cm
Originally published as Bull.no.17 of the Dept. of Agriculture under the title: The diseases and enemies of poultry

PEARSON, Robert

490 Every man his own horse, cattle, and sheep doctor; or a practical treatise on the diseases of horses, horned cattle, and sheep ... / by Robert Pearson. — Leicester: Printed for the author by J. Browne and may be had of Mr. Blanchard ..., 1811. — xxvii, [1] (blank), 428p; 22cm (8vo)
Errata leaf inserted after p. [xxviii]
Imperfect: t.p. missing and supplied in photocopy; p.419-428 missing

PECK, W.

491 Veterinary medicine, and therapeutics: containing the effects of medicines on various animals; the symptoms, causes, and treatment of diseases ... / by W. Peck. — London: Sold by Newman and Co. ... Thomas and Hunsley, Doncaster; and every other bookseller in town and country, 1814. — vi, [2], 175p, [2] leaves of plates (1 folded); 21cm (8vo)
Interleaved copy

PERCIVALL, William, 1792-1854
492 A series of elementary lectures on the veterinary art: wherein the anatomy, physiology, and pathology of the horse, are essayed on the general principles of medical science / by Veterinary Surgeon Percivall. — London: Longman, Hurst, Rees, Orme, and Brown, 1823-1826. — 3v (xxxvi, 377, [2]; vii, [1], 559, [1]; [iii]-vii, [1], 502p); 22cm (8vo)
Statement of responsibility on v.2 & 3: by William Percivall. Vol.1 by John Percivall(?)
Reference: Smith, III, 173

PERKS, William
493 A new treatise on farriery: pointing out the errors now in practice for the prevention of diseases in horses ... / by William Perks ... — Birmingham: Printed by Pearson and Rollason, 1783. — [12], 268, [8]p; 19cm (12mo)
Subscribers' list: p.[5-12]
Reference: Smith, II, 139-140

PHYSICIAN
494 An essay in order to fix the nature and cure of the distemper now raging among the horned cattle: addressed to the justices of the peace ... / by a physician. — Lincoln: Printed and sold by J.Rose ..., [1747?]. — v, [6]-14+p; 20cm (4to)
Imperfect: lacking all after p.14 (B3). Bound with: Five hundred points of good husbandry / by Thomas Tusser. — London: T.R. & M.D. for the Company of Stationers, 1672 (Copy 2)

PHYSIOLOGUS, Philotheos
see TRYON, Thomas, 1634-1703

PIPER, Hugh
495 Poultry: a practical guide to the choice, breeding, rearing and management of all descriptions of fowls, turkeys, guinea-fowls, ducks and geese for profit and exhibition / by Hugh Piper. — 2nd ed. — London: Groombridge & Sons, 1872. — vii, [1], 152p, [8] leaves of plates: col.ill; 19cm

PLAT, Sir Hugh, 1552-1611?
496 The jevvel house of art and nature: containing divers rare and profitable inventions, together with sundry new experiments in the art of husbandry ... / by Sir Hugh Plat ...; wherunto is added, A rare and excellent discourse of minerals, stones, gums and rosins; with the vertues and use thereof. By D.B. Gent. — London: Printed by Bernard Alsop ..., 1653. — [8], 232p: ill; 19cm (4to)
D.B. is Arnold Boate. Cf.DNB v.45, p.408
Reference: Wing P2390

497 The **POCKET FARRIER:** and ten minutes' advice to the purchasers of horses. — A new ed. with observations and receipts for the cure of most distempers incident to dogs. — London: Houlston & Wright, [18--]. — 36, [3]-36p: ill; 14cm. — (Houlston & Wright's industrial library)

The engraved frontispiece plate The age of a horse by its teeth in this Pocket farrier appears to have been re-drawn from that in Multum in parvo by William Taplin (615)

The **POCKET FARRIER, OR APPROVED RECEIPTS**
see FORESTER, Brooke

POTTS, Thomas, 1778-1842

498 The British farmer's cyclopaedia: being a new & complete agricultural dictionary of improved modern husbandry / by Thomas Potts. — Second edition. — London: Printed for J. Baxter, Lewes & Chichester & B. Crosby & Co. ..., 1809. — [632]p, [43] leaves of plates: ill (some col.); 28cm (4to)
Engraved t.p., followed by t.p. of 1st ed.
Signatures: [A]-4K4

499 **POULTRY AS A MEAT SUPPLY**: being hints to hen-wives how to rear and manage poultry economically and profitably / by the author of the "Poultry Kalendar". — 4th ed. — Edinburgh: William P. Nimmo, 1866. — 144p; 17cm

500 The **POULTRY DOCTOR**: including the homoeopathic treatment and care of chickens, turkeys, geese, ducks and singing birds also a materia medica of the chief remedies. — Philadelphia: Boericke & Tafel, 1891. — 85p; 20cm

501 **POULTRY FARMING AS DESCRIBED BY THE WRITERS OF ANCIENT ROME** / (Cato, Varro, Columella and Palladius); with an introduction by Alessandro Ghigi. — Milano: Ministry of Agriculture and Forestry of Italy, 1939. — 108p: ill; 24cm
Published on the occasion of the 7th World's Poultry Congress, Cleveland
Parallel Latin text and English translation

502 **POULTRY FOR EXHIBITION, HOME, AND MARKET**: with a chapter on pheasants and pheasantries / by a poultry-farmer. — London: Swan Sonnenschein, Lowrey, 1888. — vi, [2], 95p, [16] leaves of plates: ill; 22cm

POWIS, R. (Richard)

503 An examination of the different systems of shoeing the feet of horses: particularly the thin-heeled system of the College ... / by R. Powis ... — London: Published by Cradock and Joy ... and sold by J. Ebers ..., 1814. — 42p; 20cm (8vo)
Disbound

PRACTICAL FARRIER

504 A complete stable directory: for the use of the gentleman, the farmer, the groom, and the farrier ... / a Practical farrier. — London: Printed for the author, and sold by James Cummings ..., 1801. — [12], 268, [8]p; 18cm (12mo)
List of subscribers: p.[5]-[12]
This anonymous work appears to be unrecorded: not in BL or NUC; not known to Smith or to Huth; not in RVC or RCVS

505 The pocket farrier: a treatise on the veterinary art; containing the materia medica and pharmacopoeia / by a Practical farrier. — London: T. Allman, [18--]. — [5]-324p, [1] leaf of plates: ill; 12cm (8vo)
Spine title: Every man his own farrier
This anonymous work consists of a digest of other authors and quotes liberally – with acknowledgements – from Clater, Richard Lawrence, White, Gibson, Feron, Blaine, Moorcroft, Wilkinson, Coleman, Goodwin, Clark, and The Veterinary College. The section Veterinary materia medica is abridged from the corresponding text by James White (Vol. II)

506 The **PRACTICAL FARRIER**: or, full instructions for country gentlemen, farmers, graziers ... / by a Society of Country Gentlemen, Farmers, Graziers, Sportsmen, &c. — The third edition. With the addition of several curious receipts. — London: Printed and sold by E. Owen ... and by T. Astley ..., 1733. — 112, [8]p; 16cm (12mo)
Bound with: The gentleman's pocket-farrier / William Burdon. — 3rd ed. — London: J. Clarke ... S. Birt ... J. Shuckburgh, 1735

507 The **PRACTICAL FARRIER**: or, full instructions for country gentlemen, farmers, graziers ... / by a Society of Country Gentlemen, Farmers, Graziers, Sportsmen, &c. — The fourth edition. With the addition of several curious receipts. — London: Printed and sold by T. Longman ... and T. Astley ..., 1737. — 91, [5]p; 16cm (12mo)
Bound with: The gentleman's pocket farrier / by Captain Burdon. – 4th ed. — London: W. Johnston, 1748
Consists of a thinly disguised reprint of the work by Burdon, The gentleman's pocket-farrier; ... (117-124) followed by the "... best receipts ..." communicated by the members of the Society, which is not identified. See Smith (II, 27) who notes an edition of 1732 (copy in RVC)

PRACTICAL SHEPHERD
508 The flock master's companion, and shepherd's guide: containing the particulars and description of the different breeds of sheep, with their treatment ... / by a Practical shepherd. — [Royston]: Royston Press: J. Warren, 1835. — xi, 72p; 19cm (12mo)
Errata slip inserted

PRICE, Daniel
509 A system of sheep-grazing and management: as practised in Romney Marsh / by Daniel Price, of Appledore, Kent. — London: Printed for Richard Phillips ... by B. McMillan ..., 1809. — viii, 487, [1]p, [1], II [i.e.XI] leaves of plates: ill, map, plans; 28cm (4to)

PRINGLE, R. O. (Robert Oliphant)
510 The diseases of horses, cattle, sheep, swine, dogs, and poultry: their causes, symptoms, and treatment / collected and arranged from the best authorities by R.O. Pringle. — 3rd ed. — Dublin: Edward Purdon, 1872. — xii, 244p; 18cm
At head of title: Purdon's veterinary hand-book

511 **PROFITS IN POULTRY**: useful and ornamental breeds and their profitable management. — New York: O. Judd Co., 1887. — 256p: ill; 19cm

512 **PROFITS IN POULTRY:** useful and ornamental breeds and their profitable management. — New York: Orange Judd Company, 1887 (1892 printing). — 256p: ill; 19cm

PROSSER, Thomas
513 A treatise on the strangles and fevers of horses: with a plate representing a horse in the staggers slung / by Thomas Prosser. — Second edition with alterations and an index. — London: Printed for B. Uphill ... [and 3 others], [1795?]. — viii, [2], 142, iv, [1]p, [1] leaf of plates: ill; 22cm (8vo)
Errata: last p.
Verso of 2nd leaf is numbered: ii

PRUDENT LE CHOYSELAT
514 [Discours oeconomique. English] A discourse of housebandrie: no lesse profitable then delectable ... / written in the Frenche tongue by Maister Prudent Choselat; and lately translated into Englishe by R.E. — Jmprinted at London by Jhon Kyngston, for Myles Jenynges ..., 1577. — [30]p; 20cm (4to)
Translator assumed to be Richard Eden
Reference: STC (2nd ed.) 20452
The first edition of the first book in English devoted to poultry, translated from the French first published in 1569. Only two other copies of this 1577 edition are recorded, both in NUC. Neither Punnett (807) nor the University of Reading (516) were aware of the 1577 edition; the English edition of 1580 is recorded only in BL (two copies) and at Rothamsted (the copy ex Harrison Weir used by Reading) apart from NUC (two copies). It is believed that the title leaf in our copy is a facsimile printed from one of the copies in the USA

515 [Discours oeconomique. English] A discourse of housebandrie: no lesse profitable then delectable ... / written in the Frenche tongue by Maister Prudens Choiselat; and lately translated into Englishe by R.E. — [London]: Imprinted ... by Jhon Kyngston for Myles Jennynges ..., 1580 ([19--] photocopy). — 1v.; 18cm
Translator assumed to be Richard Eden

516 The Discours oeconomique of Prudent Choyselat / the first book in English on poultry husbandry translated out of the French by R.E.: with a preface by H.A.D. Neville. — [Reading]: University of Reading, 1951. — ix, 31p; 22cm
Translator assumed to be Richard Eden
No. 20 of a limited edition of 200

PUNNETT, Reginald Crundall, b.1875
517 Heredity in poultry / by Reginald Crundall Punnett. — London: Macmillan, 1923. — xi, 204p, 12 leaves of plates: ill (some col.); 19cm

R., E.
The experienced farrier
see E.R.

R., J.L.
Traité des oiseaux de basse-cour et du lapin domestique
see J.L.R.

RANDALL, Henry S., 1811-1876
518 The practical shepherd: a complete treatise on the breeding, management and diseases of sheep / by Henry S. Randall. — 20th ed. — Rochester, N.Y.: D.D.T. Moore, 1864. — 454p, [1] leaf of plates: ill; 21cm

519 Sheep husbandry: with an account of the different breeds ... / by Henry S. Randall. — New York: C.M. Saxton, 1854. — 320p: ill; 23cm

RAREY, J. S. (John Solomon), 1827-1866
520 The modern art of taming wild horses / by J.S. Rarey. — Repr. from the American ed. — London: G. Routledge & Co., 1858. — 63p; 17cm

RÉAUMUR, René Antoine Ferchault de, 1683-1757
521 Art de faire éclorre et d'élever en toute saison des oiseaux domestiques de toutes espèces: soit par le moyen de la chaleur du fumier, soit par le moyen de celle du feu ordinaire / par M. de Réaumur ... — A Paris: De l'Imprimerie royale, 1749. — 2v (xii, 342p, [9] folded leaves of plates; [4], 339p, [6] folded leaves of plates): ill; 18cm (12mo)

522 [Art de faire éclorre et d'élever en toute saison des oiseaux domestiques. English] The art of hatching and bringing up domestick fowls of all kinds at any time of the year: either by means of the heat of hot-beds, or that of common fire / by M. de Reaumur ... — London: Printed for C. Davis ..., A. Millar, and J. Nourse ..., 1750. — [2], viii, 470, [1]p, 15 folded leaves of plates: ill; 21cm (8vo)
Errata: p.[471]
Translated from the French (by A. Trembley?)

The art of hatching and bringing up domestic fowls
see also TREMBLEY, Abraham, 1710-1784

523 Pratique de l'art de faire éclorre et d'élever en toute saison des oiseaux domestiques de toutes espèces: soit par le moyen de la chaleur du fumier, soit par le moyen de celle du feu ordinaire / par M. de Réaumur ... — A Paris: De l'Imprimerie royale, 1751. — xij, 144p, 4 folded leaves of plates: ill; 17cm (12mo)
The four plates have been rearranged and do not correspond with those in the full two-volume work (521)

REAY, Henry Utrick

524 A short treatise on that useful invention called the sportsman's friend; or, the farmer's footman / by a gentleman farmer, of Northumberland; with figures of the instrument and its use, engraved on wood, by Thomas Bewick ... — Newcastle: Printed by Edward Walker ... sold by R. Fauldner ... London ..., 1801. — [2], xi, [12]-24p, [3] leaves of plates: ill; 19cm (8vo)
Erratum: p.[2]
By Henry Utrick Reay. Cf. NUC pre-1956, v.483, p.554
1st p. dated June 1801

REEVES, John

525 The art of farriery: both in theory and practice ... / by Mr. John Reeves ...; the whole revised, corrected, and enlarged by a physician; to which is added a new method of curing a strain ... also an appendix ... by an eminent surgeon. — The second edition. — Salisbury: Printed by B. Collins, for J. Newbery ... and Stanley Crowder ..., London, 1763. — [8], 408p, [4] leaves of plates (1 folded): ill; 20cm (8vo)

526 The art of farriery: both in theory and practice ... / by Mr. John Reeves ... the whole revised, corrected, and enlarged by a physician; to which is added, a new method of curing a strain ... also an appendix ... by an eminent surgeon. — The fourth edition. — London: Printed for Carnan and Newbery ...; Stanley Crowder ... and B. Collins in Salisbury, 1778. — [8], 416p, [5] leaves of plates (1 folded): ill; 21cm (8vo)
The second edition of The art of farriery ... (1763) contains three whole-page and one folded plate. In the fourth edition (1778) a fifth plate of Age by the teeth, together with explanatory text page, have been added

REID, William

527 Sheep: their history, management, diseases, and national value: with remarks on the transit of stock / by William Reid. — Edinburgh: William P. Nimmo, 1871. — viii, 146, [41]p: ill; 18cm
Advertisements on [41]p at end

RENTON, George

528 The graziers' ready reckoner: or, a useful guide for buying and selling cattle ... / by George Renton ... — Seventh edition. — London: Printed for Sherwood, Neely, and Jones ..., 1818. — 39, [3]p, [1] leaf of plates: ill; 17cm (4to)

RICHARDSON, H. D.

529 Domestic fowl and ornamental poultry: their natural history, origin, and treatment in health and disease / by H.D. Richardson. — A new ed. much enl. — London: Wm. S. Orr & Co., [1851]. — [4], 160, [4]p, [1] leaf of plates: ill; 18cm. — (Richardson's rural hand-books)

530 Domestic pigs: their origin and varieties, management with a view to profit ... / by H.D. Richardson. — A new ed. much enl. — London: Wm. S. Orr & Co., [1852?]. — iv, [7]-126, [2]p, [1] leaf of plates: ill; 18cm

RINGSTED, Josiah, d. 1812

531 The cattle-keeper's assistant; or complete directory: for country gentlemen, farmers, ... / by a gentleman from 40 years experience. — Manchester: Printed by A. Swindells ... and sold by T. Thomas, and J. Sadler, [17--]. — 96p; 19cm (8vo)
Appendix from Markham's Master-piece: p. 83-88
By J. Ringsted
Pirated ed? Cf. Southampton, 1452

532 The cattle-keeper's assistant; or complete directory for country gentlemen, farmers, ... / arranged by the most celebrated cattle-breeders in the Kingdom ... to which is added, the farmer's ready-reckoner ... — Manchester: Printed and sold by A. Swindells ..., [17--]. — 96p; 19cm (8vo)
Appendix from Markham's Master-piece: p.84-88
By J. Ringsted
Pirated ed? Cf. Southampton, 1452

533 The cattle-keeper's assistant; or complete directory: for country gentlemen, sportsmen, farmers ... / by Josiah Ringsted, esq. — The seventh edition, improved and enlarged. — London: Printed for J. Dixwell ..., [177-?]. — 81, [10]p; 21cm (8vo)
Bound with: The farmer / by Josiah Ringsted. — London: Printed for J. Dixwell, [177-]

534 The farmer: comprehending the several most interesting objects and beneficial practices in the culture of wheat, rye ... / by Josiah Ringsted, esq; ... — London: Printed for J. Dixwell ..., [177-]. — vii, [8]-166, [6]p; 21cm (8vo)
Bound with: The cattle-keeper's assistant / by Josiah Ringsted. — 7th ed. — London: Printed for J. Dixwell, [177-?]

ROLAND, Arthur

535 Poultry-keeping / by Arthur Roland; edited by William H. Ablett. — London: Chapman and Hall, 1887. — vii, [2]-162p; 21cm
A catalogue of books published by Chapman & Hall, April 1889, (40p.) follows the text

ROUS, Peyton

536 Observations on chicken tumors caused by filterable agents. — [S.l.: s.n., 1920?]. — 152p, [34] leaves of plates; 26cm
A collection of reprints by Peyton Rous et al.

ROWLANDS, Thomas

537 A treatise on the disorders incident to horned cattle: comprising, description of their symptoms, and the most rational methods of cure ... / by Thomas Rowlands. — Bangor: Printed by John Broster, 1812. — [1], xi, 100p; 23cm (4to)
Subscribers names: p.[iv-v]
The text is an almost word-for-word plagiarism of the work of the same title by Downing (229-231). The half-title, title, dedication, preface, table of contents, and the first 89 pages of text are virtually identical. Only a few recipes for diseases in sheep and swine have been added. Not known to Smith; this copy ex B. Vivash Jones MRCVS

ROWLIN, Joshua, 1708-1792

538   The complete cow-doctor, or, farmer's companion: treating of the most common disorders of black-cattle – their causes, symptoms and cures / by Joshua Rowlin, of Hollins ... — Glasgow: Printed by David Niven; for R. & P. Walker, Cockermouth, and sold by G. Robinson & Co. ... [and 6 others], 1794. — [4], 275p; 21cm (8vo)

539   The complete cow-doctor; or, farmer's companion: treating of the most common disorders of black-cattle, their causes, symptoms, and cures / by Joshua Rowlin ... — The second edition. — London: Sold by G.G. and J. Robinson, and Champante and Whitrow; also by R. Walker, Macclesfield, 1799. — viii, 211p; 19cm (12mo)
Ms. note inserted

540   The complete cow-doctor, or farmer's companion: treating of the most common disorders of black-cattle, their causes, symptoms, and cures / by Joshua Rowlin ... — The sixth edition with additions. — London: Printed by Barnard and Sultzer ... for R.S. Kirby ..., [ca.1810]. — [8], 216p; 15cm (12mo)
Edited by R. Walker
Reference: Smith, II, 209
Date on spine: 1804

RUINI, Carlo

541   Anatomia del cavallo, infermita, et suoi rimedii: opera nuova ... / del sig. Carlo Ruini ... — In Venetia: Appresso Fiorauante Prati, 1618. — [4], 247, [23], 300, [17]p: ill; 34cm (fol.)
Pt.2: Infermita del cavallo et suoi rimedii has separate t.p. and pagination
Illustrations: page 16 and 130

RUSIUS, Laurentius, 1288-1347

542   Hippiatria sive marescalia / Laurentii Rusii. — Lutetiae: Apud Christianum Wechelum ..., 1532. — [8], 143p: ill; 33cm (fol.)

543   Opera de l'arte del malscalcio / di Lorenzo Rusio ... — In Venetia: Per Michele Tramezino, 1548 del mese di Aprile. — 102, [5] leaves; 15cm (8vo)
Imprint partially from colophon
Translated from the Latin by Michele Tramezino
Some p. shaved on top with loss of running title. Bound with: Della domatione del poledro. — In Vinegia: Appresso il Biondo, 1549. Provenance: J. Gomez de la Cortina (armorial bookplate)

RYDGE, John

544   The veterinary surgeon's vade mecum: a complete guide to the cure of all diseases incident to horses, cattle, sheep, and dogs ... / by John Rydge. — London: Clerc Smith, 1827. — xxii, [2], 335p, [2] leaves of plates: col. ill; 22cm (12mo)

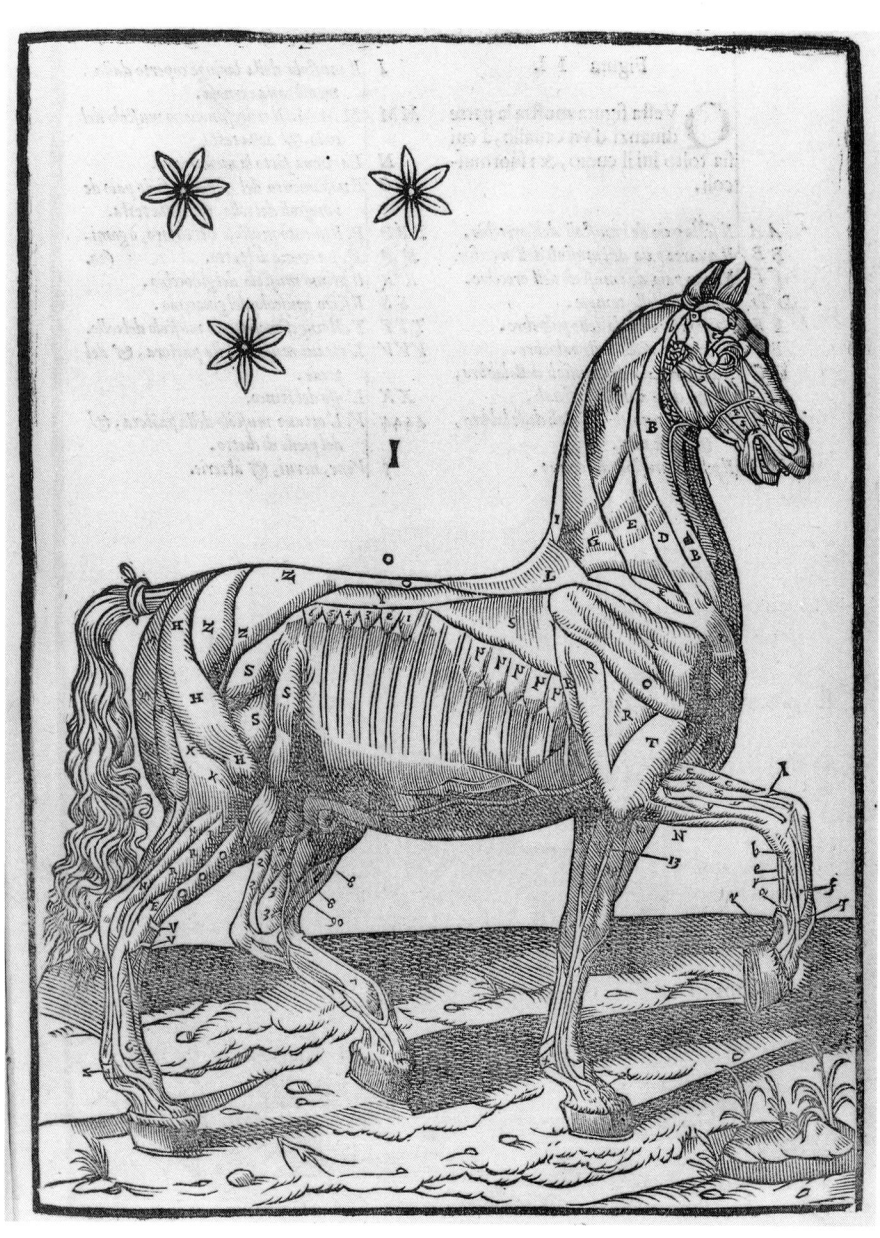

S., A.
The gentleman's compleat jockey
see A.S.

The husbandman, farmer, and grasier's compleat instructor
see A.S.

The husbandman's instructor
see A.S.

S., M.
The country-man's jewel
see M.S.

SAINBEL, Charles Vial de, 1753-1793

545 Essai sur les proportions géométrales de l'Eclipse / par M. Charles Vial de Saint Bel ... = Of the proportions of Eclipse; by Mr. Charles Vial de Saint Bel ... — London: Printed by Stephen Couchman ... and sold by Edwards and Jeffery ... [and 4 others], 1791. — viii, 67p, III folded leaves of plates: ill; 31cm (fol.)
Parallel French and English text

546 [Selections. English] The sportsman, farrier and shoeing-smiths, new guide / being the substance of the works of the late Charles Vial de St. Bell ...; to which is prefixed a short account of his life & the origin of the College. Also, an appendix, containing valuable extracts, from the most approved veterinary writers by John Lawrence, late of Lambeth Marsh, Surrey. — London: Printed for the proprietors, and sold by B. Crosby ... [and 4 others], [1796]. — iv, 232, [12]p, [1], III leaves of plates: ill; 19cm (12mo)
Engraved t.p.

547 The works of Charles Vial de Sainbel, Professor of Veterinary Medicine / to which is prefixed a short account of his life. Including also the origin of the Veterinary College of London. — London: Printed for Martin and Bain ... sold also by Mess. B. & J. White [and 4 others], 1795. — [2], 29, [1] (blank), 83, [1], 2, xii, [2], iii, [4]-202, 127, [1], 2p, [1], III, [1], IV leaves of plates (some folded): ill, port.; 27cm (4to)
Errata: on p. [xiii]
Issued without models of the hoofs and shoes (Smith, II, 197, 199-203)
Special title pages
Contents: An essay on the proportions of Eclipse — Lectures on the elements of farriery — The posthumous works
Illustration: page 132

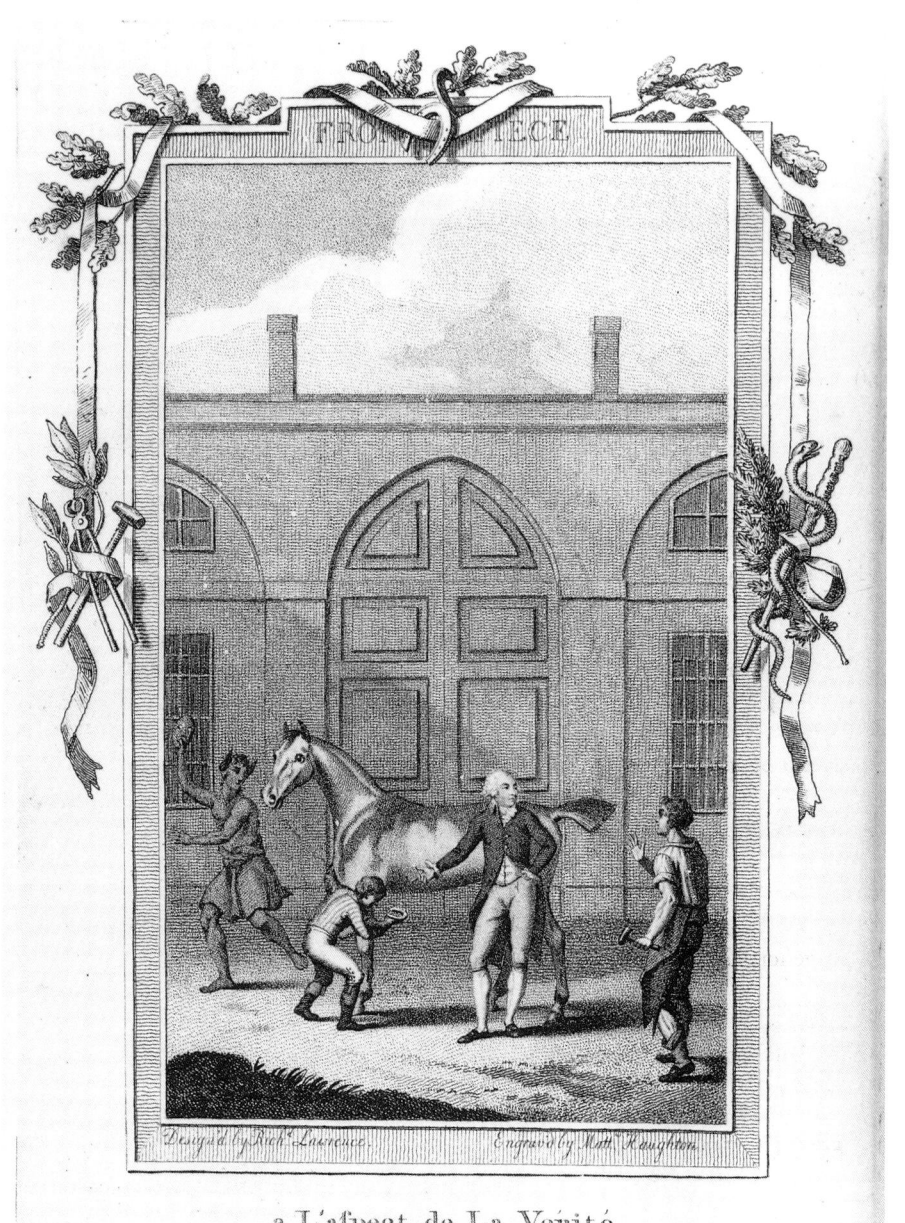

a L'aspect de La Vérité
La Routine S'etonne, L'ignorance S'enfuit.

London. Printed for Martin & Bain, Fleet Street. May 1.1795.

Sainbel 1795 (547)

SALCHOW, Ulrich Christoph, 1722-1787

548 [Durchseuchungscur] Ulrich Christoph Salchow ... erläutert und bestätiget mit noch mehrern Beyspielen, Gründen und Beobachtungen seine erfundene und bekanntgemachte untrügliche Durchseuchungscur: und zeigt zugleich die Richtschnur, nach welcher die Tilgung und gänzliche Ausrottung die Rindviehseuche bewirket werden könne. — Bremen: bey Georg Ludewig Förster, 1780. — [22], 199p: ill; 18cm (8vo)

SAUNDERS, Alfred

549 Our domestic birds: a practical poultry book for England and New Zealand / by Alfred Saunders. — London: Sampson Low, Marston, Searle & Rivington, 1883. — vi, [2], 261p: ill; 23cm

SAUNIER, Jean de

550 La parfaite connoissance des chevaux: leur anatomie, leurs bonnes & mauvaises qualitez, leurs maladies & les remèdes qui y conviennent / par J. de Saunier ...; continuée & donnée au public par son fils Gaspard de Saunier ... — A la Haye: Imprimé pour l'auteur ... et se vend chez Adrien Moetjens ..., 1734. — [8], 256, [8]p, [1], 61 leaves of plates: ill, port; 41cm (fol)

551 [Parfaite connoissance des chevaux. English] A guide to the perfect knowledge of horses: wherein every thing necessary for the choice, management and preservation of that noble and useful animal are clearly laid down ... / being the result of the long experience of that able master, M. de Saunier ... — London: Printed for W. Nicoll ... [and 3 others], 1769. — vii, [1] (blank), 272, [24]p, [9] folded leaves of plates: ill; 21cm (8vo)
French edition (1734) was edited by Gaspard de Saunier
The works of J. (father) and G. (son) de Saunier are discussed by Smith in his passage devoted to J. Brindley (II, 39-43)

La parfaite connoissance des chevaux
see also NEWCASTLE, William Cavendish, Duke of, 1592-1676
A general system of horsemanship ... Vol.II

SCOTT, Charles

552 The practice of sheep-farming / by Charles Scott. — Edinburgh: Thomas C. Jack, 1886. — xvi, [9]-210p: ill; 20cm

SCOTT, John

553 Blackfaced sheep: their history, distribution, and improvement, with methods of management and treatment of their principal diseases / by John Scott and Charles Scott. — Edinburgh: Thomas C. Jack, 1888. — xiv, [2], 307p, [5] leaves of plates: ill, port; 20cm
G.E. Fussell's copy (inscription)

554 **SCOTT'S TABLES:** calculated for farmers, graziers, butchers, millers, & bakers ... — 2nd ed. enl. — Burton-upon-Trent: Printed and sold by G. Scott, 1828. — 74p; 92mm (4to)
Illustration: page 135

[SCRIPTORES REI RUSTICAE]
555 Libri de re rustica. — Venetiis: In aedibus Aldi, et Andreae soceri, mense Maio 1514. — [34], 308 leaves; 21cm (4to)
Imprint from colophon
Reference: Adams S805
Contents: M. Catonis lib. I — M. Terentii Varronis lib. III — L. Iunii Moderati Columellae lib. XII — Eiusdem de arboribus liber ... — Palladii lib. XIIII ...

SEBRIGHT, Sir John Saunders, 1767-1846
556 The art of improving the breeds of domestic animals: in a letter addressed to the Right Hon. Sir Joseph Banks, K.B. / by Sir John Saunders Sebright, Bart. M.P. — London: Printed for John Harding ..., 1809. — 31p; 23cm (8vo)
With [4], 36p. advertisements and catalogue of Harding's books on agriculture, etc.

SHEFFIELD, John Baker Holroyd, Earl of, 1735-1821
557 Report of the Earl of Sheffield: to the meeting at Lewes Wool Fair, 26th July, 1816. — Enlarged and amended. — London: Printed and sold by Evans and Ruffy ... sold also by J. Harding ... Sherwood, Neely and Jones ... and T. Hathway, [1816]. — [2], 37p; 20cm (12mo)
Originally published in the Farmers' journal

SHELDON, J. P. (John Prince), 1841-1913
558 Dairy farming: being the theory, practice and methods of dairying / by J.P. Sheldon. — London: Cassell, [188-?]. — [8], xxii, 570p, [25] leaves of plates: ill (some col.), map, plans ; 29cm

559 Live stock in health and disease: the breeding and management of horses, cattle, sheep, goats, pigs, and poultry with chapters on dairy farming / and a full and detailed veterinary vade-mecum by A.H. Archer; edited by J. Prince-Sheldon. — London: Cassell, [1902]. — x, [1], 627p, [40] leaves of plates: ill (some col.); 28cm

560 The **SHEPHERDS' GUIDE**: being an amalgamated association comprising the following societies: the East, South, and North Fells Associations ... — Barnard Castle: Printed by Harry Ward, 1919. — ix, 656p: ill; 19cm

SCOTT'S TABLES,

Calculated for

FARMERS, GRAZIERS, BUTCHERS, MILLERS, & BAKERS,

Shewing at one view, the Value of

CATTLE

And other Beasts, of different weights and prices, per Quarter, with a Table equalizing the weights by which they are bought and sold;

ALSO OF WHEAT

And other Grain, per bushel, of various weights;

At the same time, shewing the

COMPARATIVE VALUE OF THE WINCHESTER AND IMPERIAL BUSHEL;

And an easy correct method of ascertaining uniformity

IN WEIGHTS AND MEASURES;

Together with a Table shewing the difference between Short and Long Weight, and Long and Short Weight, from One to Twenty Hundred, and from Two to One Hundred Tons; with various other useful Tables.

Second Edition Enlarged.

BURTON-UPON-TRENT:

Printed & Sold by G. Scott, High-Street; Baldwin and Cradock, London; and all other Booksellers.

1828.

Entered at Stationers' Hall.--- Price 2s. bound.

561 The **SHEPHERD'S GUIDE**; or a delineation of the wool and ear marks of the different stocks of sheep: in Patterdale, Netherwasdale, Borrowdale, Loweswater, Kenniside ... — Penrith: Printed by W. Stephen, [1819]. — [4], 381p: chiefly ill; 20cm (4to)
Markings by hand. Imperfect: some loss of ill. on p.235 & 347
Shepherd's Guides are books which illustrate the unique 'lug' (ear marks) and 'smit' (coloured marks on the fleece) which identify sheep flocks and hence the farms to which they belong. This was the first of such Guides, collected by Joseph Walker of Martindale and published in 1819; very few copies have survived. The sheep – three to a page – are shown in outline standing facing left and right so that the marks of both sides can be illustrated. Each entry had to be hand coloured. Further Guides for the Cumberland and Westmoreland areas have been published at intervals since (in 1849, 1870, 1913, 1927, 1937, and as recently as 1985) and similar Guides for other areas (as 402-403)
Illustration: page 137

SHERER, John, b.1810
562 Rural life: described and illustrated, in the management of horses, dogs, cattle, sheep, pigs, poultry ... / by John Sherer. — London: London Printing and Publishing Co., [1868-1869]. — xvi, 1016p, [65] leaves of plates: ill; 28cm
This copy is bound in two volumes, the printed title has been bound in as a title page to the second volume. The 65 leaves of plates, which are all black and white engravings, are as follows: v.1: frontispiece and engraved title and 43 plates (of which three are folded); v.2: frontispiece and 19 plates

SHIPP, John
563 Cases in farriery: in which the diseases of horses are treated on the principles of the Veterinary School of Medicine / by John Shipp ... — Leeds: Printed by Edward Baines, for the author; and sold by Longman and Co. ... [and 6 others], [1806]. — [4], vii, [8]-237, [1] (blank), v p, [1] leaf of plates: ill; 27cm (4to)
List of subscribers: p. [i-ii]. Last leaf bound upside down

SILLETT, John
564 A practical treatise on feeding & fattening pigs ... also a report of successful experiments in the cultivation and cropping of two acres of land / by John Sillett. — London: Simpkin, Marshall, and Co., 1851. — [4], 26p: ill; 22cm
Imperfect: frontispiece missing

SIMONDS, James B., 1810-1904
565 A practical treatise on variola ovina, or small-pox in sheep: containing the history of its recent introduction into England ... / by James B. Simonds. — London: James Ridgway, 1848. — viii, 157, [1]p, 5 leaves of plates: col.ill; 25cm (4to)

SIMPSON, Pinder
566 On the improved beet root, as winter food for cattle / [by Pinder Simpson]. — London: Printed for Taylor and Hessey ..., 1814. — xvi, [17]-46p; 17cm (12mo)
Half title: On the improved beet root, or mangel wurzel
Dedication signed by Pinder Simpson

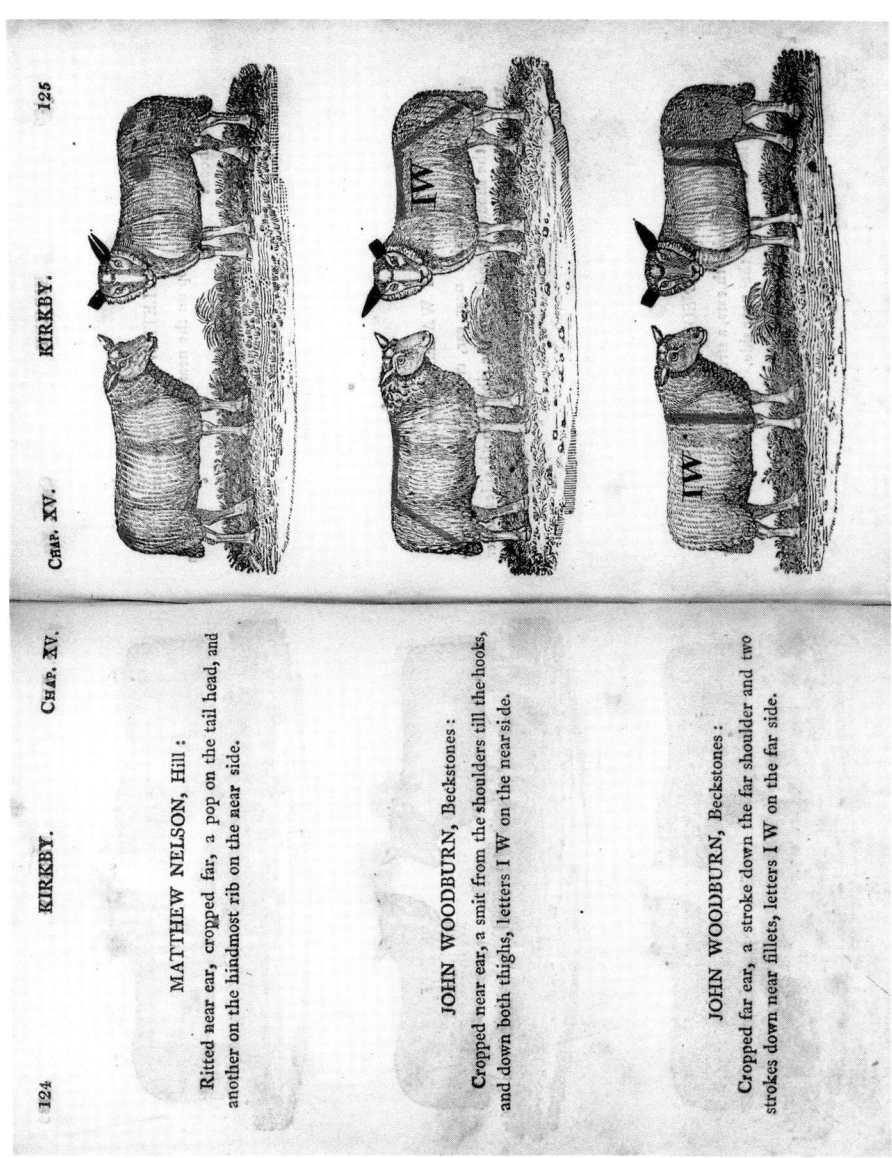

MATTHEW NELSON, Hill:

Ritted near ear, cropped far, a pop on the tail head, and another on the hindmost rib on the near side.

JOHN WOODBURN, Beckstones:

Cropped near ear, a smit from the shoulders till the hooks, and down both thighs, letters I W on the near side.

JOHN WOODBURN, Beckstones:

Cropped far ear, a stroke down the far shoulder and two strokes down near fillets, letters I W on the far side.

SINCLAIR, A. G.
567 Critical observations and remarks, on A stable directory, or, modern system of farriery, of W. Taplin ... / by A.G. Sinclair ... — London: Printed for the author, 1792. — vi, 7-80p; 29cm (4to)
Catchword on p.80: Letter
Ms. note at end: "... Taplin was glad to silence Dr. Sinclair by buying off his further corrections & admonitions". Imperfect: 1st leaf missing
Illustration: page 139

SIND, J. B., Freiherr von, 1709-1776
568 A description of the virtues and uses of a preservative electary against the glanders in horses / invented and made by the Baron de Sind ... to which is added, the verbal process of the experiments, that was made at Popplesdorff, near Bonn, by order of the French king ... — London: Printed for G. Woodfall ..., 1764. — [2] (last blank), xxi, [1] (blank), 33p; 21cm (8vo)
Noted by Huth but not otherwise recorded. Not in BL or NUC; not known to Smith; not in RVC, RCVS, or the Anderhub sale. Mennessier de la Lance notes an edition in French, 1778, and states that Sind's electuary treatment was officially tried out in France but found to be ineffective. Ex D.J. Spark

SKELLETT, Edward
569 A practical treatise on the breeding cow: and extraction of the calf ... / by Edward Skellett. — London: Sherwood, Gilbert, and Piper, [1829?]. — xi, [1], 364p, 13 folded leaves of plates: col.ill; 26cm (8vo)

570 A practical treatise on the parturition of the cow, or the extraction of the calf: and on the diseases of neat cattle in general ... / by Edward Skellett. — London: Stereotyped and printed by and for A. Wilson, 1811. — xi, [1], 364p, 13 folded leaves of plates: ill; 27cm (8vo)

SMALL, Matthew
571 Small's veterinary tablet: being a synopsis of the diseases of horses, cattle, and dogs, with their cause, symptoms, and cure / by Matthew Small. — 2nd ed. — Glasgow: W.R. M'Phun, [18--]. — 1 sheet: ill; 65x44cm folded to 18x10cm
Mounted and cased

SMART, Andrew
572 Reports to the Lord Provost and Magistrates of the City of Edinburgh on the pathological appearances, symptoms, treatment, and means of preventing cattle plague / [by Andrew Smart]. — Edinburgh: Maclachlan & Stewart, 1865. — 46, 4p, IV leaves of plates: col.ill; 28cm
Reprint of the author's Rinderpest prevention, 2 leaves, bound between p.44 and 45
Andrew Smart, MD, FRCPE, was appointed by the magistrates of the City of Edinburgh to investigate the cattle plague ... prevailing among the cows in Edinburgh. He presented four reports, which appear to have been highly regarded, and also addressed the subject of the ... liability of sheep to the disease. He claimed to have discovered a successful preventive treatment. This copy in a luxurious full red morocco leather presentation binding

CRITICAL
Observations and *Remarks,*
ON
A STABLE DIRECTORY,
OR,

Modern System of FARRIERY,

of W. TAPLIN, Surgeon:

Addreſſed to the AUTHOR,

In a Series of Letters;

In which are pointed out His Errors and Ridiculous Absurdities.

With Explanations, and Definitions of All the

Diſeaſes incident to the
HORSE,

And the Modes of CURE, as Selected from the beſt Authors;

To which are Added,

Several PRESCRIPTIONS, never before publiſhed,

not only for the uſe of the Brute, but Human Species.

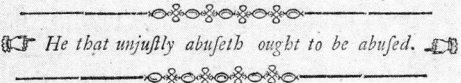

☞ *He that unjuſtly abuſeth ought to be abuſed.* ☜

By A. G. SINCLAIR, M.D.

Author of the Critic Philosopher,—Ars Medicinæ,

Comparative System of Anatomy, &c.

LONDON:

Printed for the Author, and may be had at No. 6, *Cleveland-Row*, St. *James's*.

1792.

SNAPE, Andrew, b.1644

573 The anatomy of an horse: containing an exact and full description of the frame, situation and connexion of all his parts ... to which is added an appendix, containing two discourses ... / by Andrew Snape, jun. ... — London: Printed by M. Flesher for the authour, and are to be sold by T. Flesher ..., 1683. — [12], 237, [1] (blank), 45, [6]p, XLIX leaves of plates: ill, port; 37cm (fol.)
Illustration: page 16

574 The anatomy of an horse: containing an exact and full description of the frame, situation and connexion of all his parts ... to which is added an appendix, containing two discourses ... / by Andrew Snape, jun. ... — London: Printed by M. Flesher, for J. Hindmarsh ..., 1686. — [12], 237, [1] (blank), 45, [6]p, XLIX leaves of plates: ill, port; 37cm (fol.)

575 Snape's purging pill for horses: with his cordial pouder, and ointments ... / by Andrew Snape ... — London: [s.n.], 1692. — [6], 8p; 19cm (4to)
Disbound
Andrew Snape announced his intention to write a Book of cures, but "no such work, unfortunately, saw the light" (Smith, I, 342). This copy of the pamphlet Snape's purging pill for horses: ... was discovered only in 1968. It is of particular interest as probably the first fully descriptive, printed catalogue offering animal remedies for sale – and covering the preparations, their indications and methods of use, cautions, pack sizes, storage and shelf life, prices, and distribution. Apparently unrecorded: not in BL or NUC; not known to Smith or to Huth; not in RVC or RCVS. See Comben, N. (1969) Snape's purging pill for horses – 1692. Veterinary record, 84, 434-435
Illustration: frontispiece

SNAPE, Edward

576 A practical treatise on farriery: including remarks on all diseases incident to horses ... / by Edward Snape ... — London: Printed (by H. Reynell ...) for the author ..., 1791. — [14], viii, 154, [1]p, [1] leaf of plates: port; 25cm (4to)
Errata: last p.

577 A practical treatise on farriery: including remarks on all diseases incident to horses ... / from the manuscripts of the late Edward Snape ... — London: Printed by H. Reynell ... sold by T. Ostell ... [and 3 others], 1805. — [12], viii, 152, [1]p, [1] leaf of plates: port; 28cm (4to)

SOLLEYSEL, Jacques de, 1617-1680

578 Le parfait maréchal: qui enseigne a connoître la beauté, la bonté et les défauts des chevaux ... / par le Sieur de Solleysel ... — Nouvelle édition, augmentée d'un abregé de l'art de monter à cheval. — A Paris: Chez Didot ... [and 3 others], 1754. — [6], 512, [10], 406, [2]p, [3] leaves of plates (2 folded): ill; 26cm (4to)
Additional engraved t.p.

579 [Parfait mareschal. English] The compleat horseman: discovering the surest marks of the beauty, goodness, faults and imperfections of horses ... / by the Sieur de Solleysell ...; to which is added, a most excellent supplement of riding ... by Sir William Hope ... — London: Printed for M. Gillyflower ... [and 9 others], 1696. — [52], 261, [5], 86, [18], 300, [4]p, [3], 6 folded leaves of plates : ill, port; 31cm (fol.)
Additional engraved t.p. to pt.1; engraved t.p. to pt.2

580 [Parfait mareschal. English. Selections] The compleat horseman: or, perfect farrier: in two parts ... / written in French by the Sieur de Solleysell ...; abridged from the folio done into English by Sir William Hope; with the addition of several excellent receipts, by our best farriers: and directions to the buyers and sellers of horses. — London: Printed for H. Bonwicke ... [and 4 others], 1702. — [16], 376, [16]p, [7] leaves of plates (6 folded): ill; 20cm (8vo)
Translation of: Le parfait mareschal
A compendious treatise of the art of riding, 1701, p.[183]-224 has separate t.p.

SOMERVILLE, John, 15th Baron, 1765-1819

581 Facts and observations relative to sheep, wool, ploughs, and oxen: in which the importance of improving the short-woolled breeds by a mixture of the Merino blood is deduced ... / by John, Lord Somerville. — London: Printed for William Miller ..., 1803. — viii, 137, [3]p, [3] folded leaves of plates: ill; 22cm (8vo)
Errata: p.[1] at end
Bound with: A view of the policy of Sir George Barlow / by Indus. — London: J.Ridgway, 1810 and A treatise on watering meadows. — 3rd ed. — Dublin: J. Moore, 1792

582 Facts and observations relative to sheep, wool, ploughs, and oxen: in which the importance of improving the short-wooled breeds of sheep by a mixture of the Merino blood is demonstrated ... / by John Lord Somerville. — Third edition enlarged. — London: Printed for John Harding ..., 1809. — [8], 256p, [10] leaves of plates (3 folded): ill; 22cm (8vo)
Errata: p.256
Publisher's 36p catalogue is bound at the end

583 The system followed during the two last years by the Board of Agriculture: further illustrated ... / by John, Lord Somerville. — A second edition ... — London: Printed for W. Miller ... by E. Cox & Son ..., 1800. — [4], 300, [4]p, VI [i.e. 8] folded leaves of plates: ill; 22cm (8vo)

SONNINI DE MANONCOURT, C. S. (Charles Nicolas Sigisbert), 1751-1812

584 A treatise on the breeding, rearing, and fattening of poultry: chiefly translated from the new French dictionary on natural history. — London: Printed by R. Juigné ..., 1810. — [6], 196p; 22cm (4to)
"Chiefly translated" from: Vocabulaire portatif ... / Sonnini de Manoncourt, Veillard and Chevalier

585 A treatise on the breeding, rearing, and fattening of poultry. — 2nd ed. — London: Printed for James Ridgway, 1819. — [6], 196p; 21cm (4to)
Colophon reads: R. Juigné, printer ...
Translated from: Vocabulaire portatif ... / Sonnini de Manoncourt, Veillard and Chevalier

SPEED, Ad.

586 Adam out of Eden: or, an abstract of divers excellent experiments touching the advancement of husbandry ... / by Ad. Speed. gent. — London: Printed for Henry Brome ..., 1659. — [6], 163 [i.e.179], [3]p; 15cm (8vo)
Author variously as Adam or Adolphus Speed. Cf. Wing S4877; BLC
Error in pagination: p.179 as 163
Imperfect: mutilated with slight loss of text

SPILSBURY, Francis

587 Discursory thoughts, &c.: disputing the constructions of His Majesty's hon. commissioners and crown lawyers, relative to the medicine and horse acts ... / by Francis Spilsbury. — The second edition. — London: Sold at the Dispensary, in Soho Square, 1785. — [2], 53p; 20cm (8vo)
Disbound

SPOONER, W. C. (William Charles), 1809?-1885

588 The history, structure, economy, and diseases of the sheep / by W.C. Spooner; illustrated ... by W. Harvey. — London: Cradock, 1844. — xiii, 466p: ill; 19cm (12mo)
Additional engraved t.p.

589 A treatise on the influenza of horses: showing its nature, symptoms, causes, and treatment ... / by William Charles Spooner. — 2nd ed. — London: Simpkin; Southampton: Best and Snowden, 1843. — [v]-xii, 131p; 20cm (12mo)
"With an appendix containing a full account of the influenza of 1840"

590 A treatise on the structure, functions, and diseases of the foot and leg of the horse: comprehending the comparative anatomy of these parts in other animals ... / by W.C. Spooner. — London: Longman, Orme, Brown, Green and Longmans, 1840. — xx, 337p: ill; 18cm (8vo)
List of subscribers: p.[xix]-xx

591 Veterinary art: a practical treatise on the diseases of the horse / by W.C. Spooner. — 2nd ed., reprinted from the edition of 1845. — London: John Joseph Griffin & Co., 1851. — x, 107, [5]p, IV folded leaves of plates: ill; 20cm. — (Encyclopaedia metropolitana. 2nd division. Applied sciences)

592 The **SPORTSMAN AND VETERINARY RECORDER.** — London: Published at the office, 19 Old Boswell Court, Strand, 1835. — 25cm (4to)
Holdings: Vol.1 (Jan-June 1835) — v.2 (July-Dec. 1835)

593 The **SPORTSMAN'S DICTIONARY**: or, the country gentleman's companion: in all rural recreations ... / extracted from the most celebrated English and French authors, ancient, and modern ... — The second edition. — London: Printed for J. Osborn ..., 1744. — [742]p, 25, [1] leaves of plates (17 folded): ill; 21cm (8vo)

594 The **SPORTSMAN'S DICTIONARY**; or, the gentleman's companion: for town and country ... / collected from the best authors; with very considerable additions and improvements, by experienced gentlemen. — The third edition. — London: Printed for G.G.J. and J. Robinson ..., 1785. — [552]p, XVI leaves of plates: ill; 27cm (4to)

ST. JOHN, Sir Paulet
595 Every man his own farrier: being a collection of valuable and efficacious receipts, for most disorders incident to horses / carefully collected and applied with repeated success, for upwards of fifty years past, by Sir Paulet St. John, Bart. ... — Winton: Printed by J. Wilkes, and sold by S. Crowder ..., 1780. — viii, 80, [8]p; 20cm (8vo)

ST. RAPHAEL MILLING CO.
596 Price list of general farm and poultry appliances July, 1934 / St. Raphael Milling Co. — Bristol: St. Raphael Milling Co., 1934. — 102p: ill; 20cm
Cover title

STEPHENS, Henry, 1795-1874
597 The book of the farm: detailing the labours of the farmer, farm-steward, ploughman ... / by Henry Stephens. — Edinburgh; London: William Blackwood and Sons, 1844. — 3v (xix, 670p, [17] leaves of plates; [6], 728p, [16] leaves of plates; vi, 729-1407, [1]p): ill; 24cm (8vo)
Vol. 1: plates I-XVII; v.2: plates XVIII-XXXIII
Provenance: Earl of Kintore (armorial bookplate)

STEVENSON, John
598 The sportsman's, farmer's and cattle-doctor's vade mecum: containing the most approved methods ... / by John Stevenson. — London: Sherwood, Gilbert, and Piper, 1830. — xv, 189p, [1] folded leaf of plates: ill; 18cm (12mo)

STEWART, Henry
599 The shepherd's manual: a practical treatise on the sheep. Designed especially for American shepherds / by Henry Stewart. — New ed. – rev. and enl. — New York: Orange Judd, 1883. — 264p: ill; 19cm

STUBBS, George, 1724-1806
600 The anatomy of the horse: including a particular description of the bones, cartilages, muscles, fascias, ligaments, nerves, arteries, veins, and glands ... / by George Stubbs, painter. — London: Printed by J. Purser, for the author, 1766. — [4], 47p, XV [i.e.24] leaves of plates: ill; 45x56cm (double fol.)

(cont.)

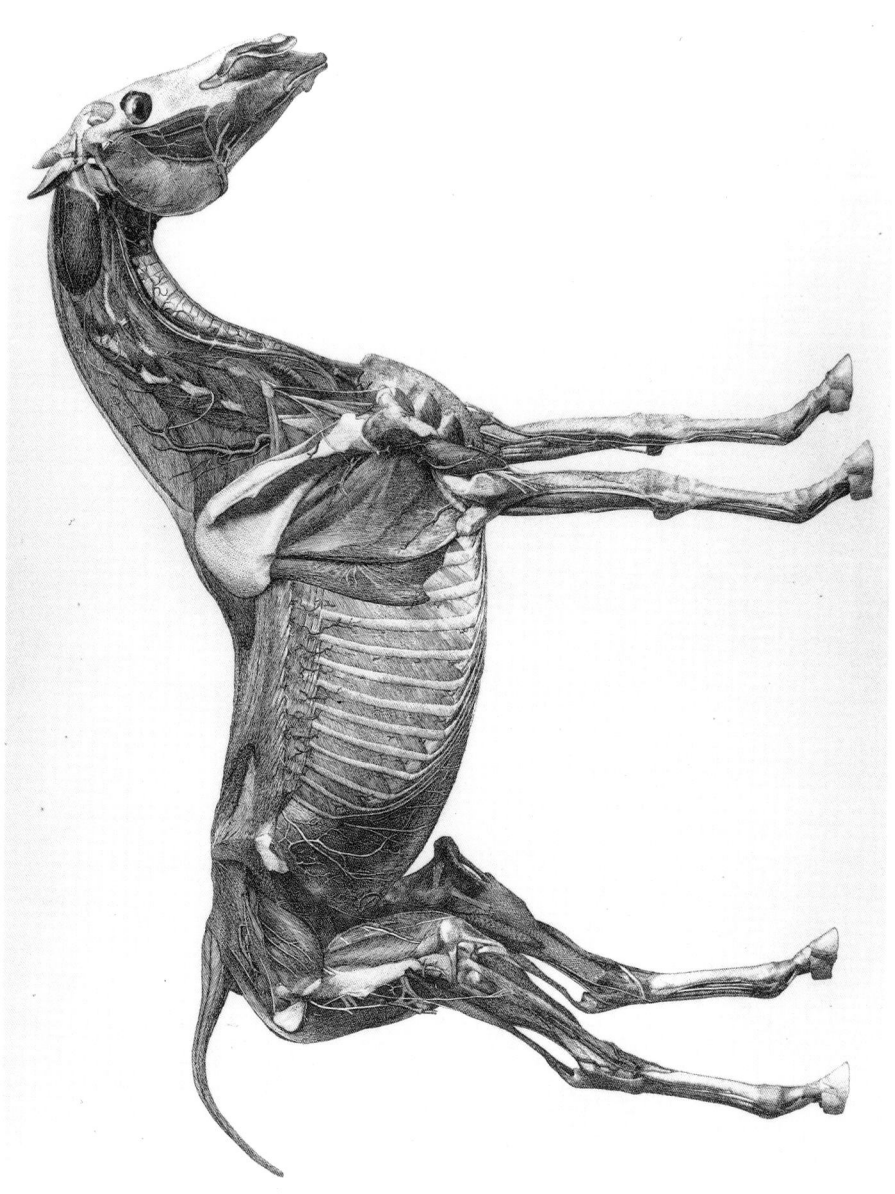

Plates watermarked 1823
Stubbs's work was first published as a landscape folio, with an errata leaf, in 1766; many copies have no watermarks. Copies of this first edition are however found with the plates printed on paper with later watermarks, certainly 1793, 1812 and 1823 (in some copies together with the text leaves watermarked 1766); such copies appear to have been made up from an original stock of text sheets, with additional plates printed as required. Subsequent English editions were in an upright folio; a second edition by Bohn in 1853, a third edition by Gibbings and Co.in 1899, a fourth edition by Heywood Hill in 1938, and various more recent editions. A quarto edition in French, translated by 'M.G.', was published in London in 1797
Illustration: page 144

STUMPF, Georg, 1750-1798
601 An essay on the practical history of sheep in Spain: and of the Spanish sheep in Saxony, Anhalt Dessau, &c. / by George Stumpf ...; translated from the German by the Rev. Dr. Lanigan ... — Dublin: Printed by Graisberry & Campbell ..., 1800. — [4], 101, [6], 104-300p, [9] leaves of plates: ill; 22cm (8vo). — (Transactions of the Dublin Society)
This volume published by the Royal Dublin Society contains, with near continuous pagination, a number of works: the translation by the Rev. Dr Lanigan of the original German text by Stumpf published in Leipzig, 1785; Extracts from the Foreign communications to the Board of Agriculture in London – Volume I; Extracts from the work in French by Daubenton, 1810 (213), reproducing Plates III-IX, XXI and XXII re-drawn from the original; and a miscellany of other contributions, on Mines (by Kirwan) and others. Copy noted in Rothamsted, but not known to Smith or to Fussell, not in RVC, RCVS or Southampton

SUTHERLAND, W.
602 "Sheep farming". A treatise on sheep: their management and diseases / by W. Sutherland. — Berkhamsted: William Cooper & Nephews, 1892. — vii, 163, [25]p, [18] leaves of plates: ill; 18cm
Advertisements on [25]p at end

SUTTON, C. W.
603 Hand-book of veterinary practice: containing the symptoms and treatment of most of the diseases ... / by C.W. Sutton. — 2nd ed. — Stowmarket: Published by the author; London: G.F. Sutton & Co., 1875. — [4], 68p; 21cm

SWAINE, John
604 Every farmer his own cattle doctor: containing, a full and clear account of the symptoms and causes of the diseases of cattle ... / by John Swaine ... — London: Printed for Richardson and Urquhart ..., [1776]. — [2], 179, [9]p; 19cm (12mo)

605 Every farmer his own cattle-doctor: containing a full and clear account of thesymptoms and causes of the diseases of cattle ... / by John Swaine ... — The third edition, with additions. — London: Printed for W. Richardson ..., 1786. — xii, 189p; 19cm (12mo)

TAM, Franz Joseph, Freiherr von

606 In danknehmigst- pflichtmässiger Liebe immergrünend entsprossenes vierfaches Kleeblatt: worin mit erwiesenen Beyspielen bestätigte 300 Hilfsmittel für Horn- Schaf- Pferd- und Federvieh ... — Wien und Prag: Gedruckt bey Johann Thomas von Trattner ..., 1764. — [26], 605p, [3] leaves of plates (2 folded): ill; 20cm (8vo)
Errata: p.602-605
Dedication signed: Franz Joseph Freyherr v. Tam
Contains a folded plate depicting various sizes of stillet for surgical procedures on sheep

TAPLIN, William, 1740?-1807

607 A compendium of practical and experimental farriery: originally suggested by reason and confirmed by practice ... / by William Taplin ... — Brentford: Printed by P. Norbury for G.G. and J. Robinson ... and G. Kearsley ..., 1796. — xi, [1], 274, [2]p, [2] leaves of plates: ill; 21cm (8vo)
Includes index

608 A compendium of practical and experimental farriery: originally suggested by reason and confirmed by practice ... / by William Taplin ... — Dublin: Printed by John Barlow, for P. Wogan [and 5 others], 1796. — x, 261, [1]p: ill; 21cm (8vo)
Two copies: one bound with: The gentleman's stable directory / by William Taplin. — Dublin: Printed for P. Wogan ... and P. Byrne ..., 1793
The Compendium ... contained a frontispiece plate of Taplin's equestrian receptacle and operative farriery (in the Edgeware Road, London) and a plate of Taplin's pattern shoes. The frontispiece plate was not issued with the Dublin edition, for which the plate of shoes was re-drawn

609 The gentleman's stable directory; or, modern system of farriery: comprehending the present entire improved mode of practice ... / by William Taplin ... — [London]: Printed for G. Kearsley ..., 1788. — xvi, 356, [12]p; 22cm (8vo)
Last [4]p are advertisements
Bound with: Practical observations upon thorn wounds, punctured tendons, and ligamentary lameness in horses / by William Taplin. — London: Printed for G. Kearsley, 1790

610 The gentleman's stable directory; or, modern system of farriery: comprehending the present entire improved mode of practice ... / by William Taplin ... — The third edition, corrected. — London: Printed for G. Kearsley ..., 1788. — xvi, 356, [12]p; 22cm (8vo)
An engraved portrait of Taplin was introduced as a frontispiece to The gentleman's stable directory ... in 1790. Vol. 2 was first published in 1791. The editions published in Dublin were produced in a smaller format in 12mo

611 The gentleman's stable directory; or, modern system of farriery: volume the second ... / by William Taplin. — London: Printed for G. Kearsley ..., 1791. — viii, 419, [5]p; 22cm (8vo)

612 [The gentleman's stable directory] For the draft, road, field, or turf. The gentleman's stable directory: or modern system of farriery: comprehending the present entire improved mode of practice ... / by William Taplin ... — The ninth edition, considerably enlarged and carefully corrected. — London printed; Dublin reprinted: by W. Wilson ... sold also by T. White, Cork; Watson & Co. Limerick; and J. and W. Magee, Belfast, 1790. — [3], xvi, 395p; 19cm (12mo)

613 [The gentleman's stable directory] For the draft, road, field, or turf. The gentleman's stable directory: or modern system of farriery: comprehending the present entire improved mode of practice: volume the second ... / by William Taplin ... — London printed; Dublin reprinted: by W. Wilson ... sold also by T. White, Cork; Watson & Co. Limerick; and J. and W. Magee, Belfast, 1791. — viii, 320p; 18cm (12mo)

614 The gentleman's stable directory: or, modern system of farriery: comprehending all the most valuable prescriptions and approved remedies ... / by William Taplin ... — The eleventh edition, with very considerable additions. — Dublin: Printed for P. Wogan ... and P. Byrne ..., 1793. — 2v. in 1 (xxiii, [1], 255p, 4 leaves of plates; viii, 191p): ill; 20cm (8vo)
The four plates, which were not published with the London editions of this work, have been plagiarised from Gibson
Vol. 2 is: The third edition, carefully corrected
Bound with: A compendium of practical and experimental farriery / by William Taplin. — Dublin: Printed by John Barlow, for P. Wogan [and 5 others], 1796 (copy 2)

615 [Multum in parvo] Taplin's Multum in parvo. Or Sportsmans equestrian monitor. — London: Printed for the author ... and sold by J.Wheble ..., 1796. — [2], viii, [9]-104p, [2] leaves of plates: ill; 17cm (8vo)
List of subscribers: p.93-97
Not seen by Smith
Illustration: page 148

616 Practical observations upon thorn wounds, punctured tendons, and ligamentary lameness in horses: with experimental instructions for their treatment and cure ... the whole forming a supplement to The gentleman's stable directory / by William Taplin ... — London: Printed for G. Kearsley ..., 1790. — 88p; 22cm (8vo)
Bound with: The gentleman's stable directory / by William Taplin. — [London]: G. Kearsley, 1788

617 Taplin improved; or, a compendium of farriery: wherein is fully explained the nature and structure of that useful creature, a horse ... / by an experienced farrier. — London: Printed by H. Harrison, for N. Frobisher ... York, 1790. — v (i.e.iv), [5]-144p, [8] folded leaves of plates: ill; 14cm (18mo)
Vertical chain lines

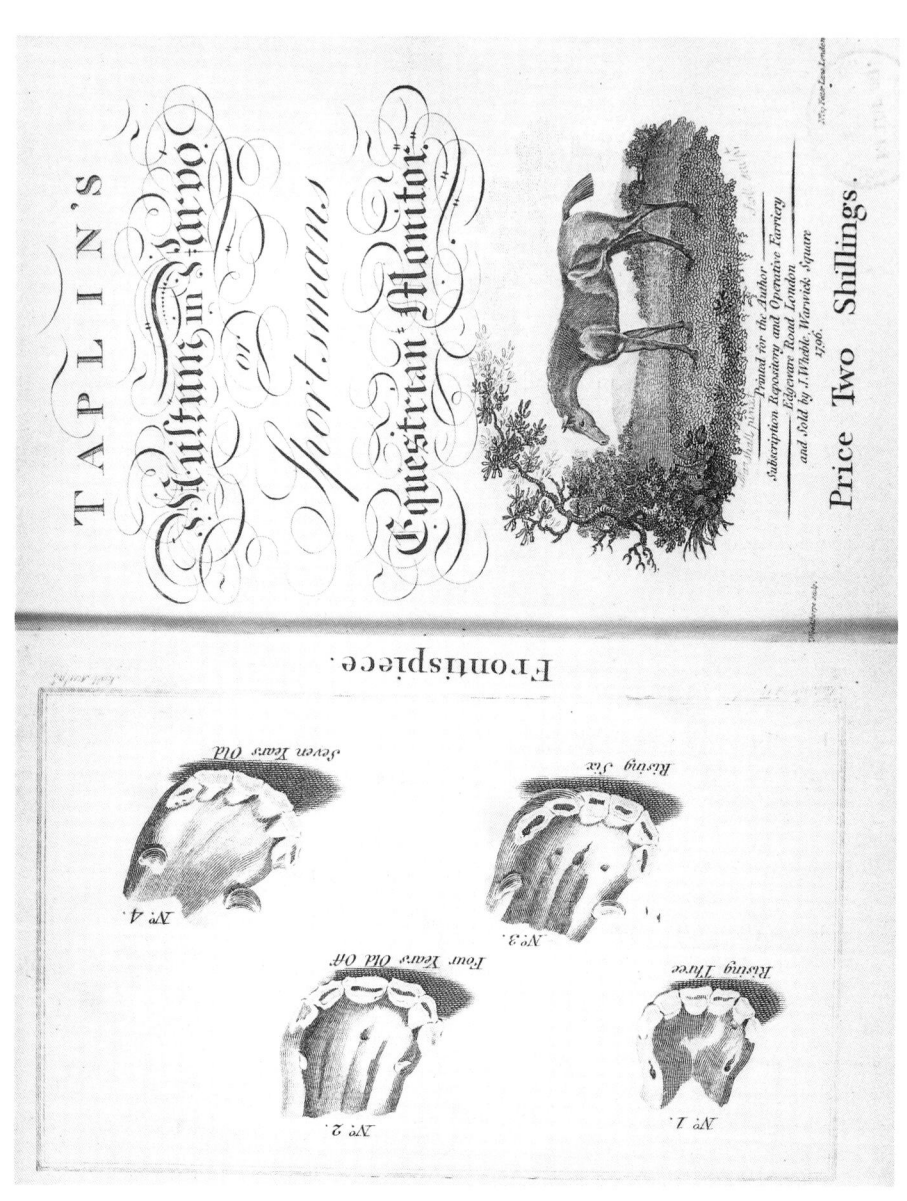

618 Taplin improved; or a compendium of farriery: wherein is fully explained the nature and structure of that useful creature a horse ... / by an experienced farrier. — London: Printed for William Lane, at the Minerva=Press ..., 1794. — 144p, 10 leaves of plates: ill; 16cm (12mo)

619 Taplin improved; or a compendium of farriery: wherein is fully explained the nature and structure of that useful creature a horse ... / by an experienced farrier. — London: Printed for William Lane, at the Minerva=Press ..., 1796. — iv, [5]-144p, 10 leaves of plates: ill; 17cm (12mo)

620 Taplin improved; or a compendium of farriery: wherein is fully explained the nature and structure of that useful creature a horse ... / by an experienced farrier. — London: Printed for B. Crosby and Co. ... W. Norman, printer, Aylesbury, 1807. — iv, [5]-135, [9]p, 10 leaves of plates: ill; 16cm (12mo)

621 Taplin improved: or, a compendium of farriery: wherein is fully explained the nature and structure of that useful creature, a horse ... / by an experienced farrier. — London: Printed for B. Crosby and Co. ... by John Jackson, Louth, 1811. — v, [6]-144p, 10 leaves of plates: ill; 16cm (12mo)
The five works issued under the title Taplin improved ... are plagiarisms for which Taplin was not responsible (see Smith, II, 163 & 173). The two Lane's and two Crosby's editions contain the same frontispiece plate of a horseman with a prancing horse; this is not present in the 1790 edition. All editions have plates copied and re-drawn from de Saunier (551). The texts contain material on The cure of sheep and lambs, hogs, and dogs, and on destroying moles, subjects not covered in Taplin's own works. (See also, Bracken, 98)

TEGETMEIER, W. B. (William Bernhard), 1816-1912

622 Pigeons: their structure, varieties, habits, and management / by W.B. Tegetmeier; with coloured representations of the different varieties drawn from life by Harrison Weir. — London: G. Routledge and Sons, [1873?]. — [4], 190p, [16] leaves of plates: col.ill; 29cm

623 The poultry book: comprising the breeding and management of profitable and ornamental poultry to which is added "The standard of excellence in exhibition birds" / by W.B. Tegetmeier; with coloured illustrations by Harrison Weir. — New ed. — London: George Routledge and Sons, 1873. — viii, 390p, [30] leaves of plates: col.ill; 29cm

624 Profitable poultry: their management in health and disease / by W.B. Tegetmeier. — New ed. greatly enl. — London: Darton and Co., 1854. — 48p, [4] leaves of plates: col.ill; 19cm

TESSIER, H.-A. (Henri-Alexandre), 1741-1837

625 Instruction sur les bêtes à laine: et particulièrement sur la race des mérinos ... / rédigée par M. Tessier ... — A Paris: De l'Imprimerie impériale, 1810. — 355, [1]p, [1], 6 folded leaves of plates: ill; 20cm (8vo)
Fautes à corriger: last p.

THOMPSON, Charles
626 Rules for bad horsemen: addressed to the Society for the Encouragement of Arts, &c. / by Charles Thompson, esq;. — London: Printed for J. Robson ..., 1762. — [2], iv, 82p; 17cm (8vo)
Errata: on p.82

TIBBS, Thomas
627 The experimental farmer: being strictures on various branches of husbandry and agriculture ... / by Thomas Tibbs, farmer ... — London: Printed by and for A. Kemmish ... and the author: Published by Thomas Ostell ..., 1807. — xiv, [15]-153, [10]p: 23cm (8vo)
Errata: last p.
Signed by the author. G.E. Fussell's copy (signature)
Reference: Fussell, III, 64

TINDALL, John
628 Observations on the breeding and management of neat cattle: together with a description of the diseases to which they are liable ... / by John Tindall. — Leeds: Printed for the author by Edward Baines, 1811. — [4], xi, [10]-226p, [3] leaves of plates: ill; 23cm (8vo)
Subscribers' names: [219]-226
Erratum: p.[10]

629 Observations on the breeding and management of neat cattle: with descriptions of the diseases to which they are liable ... / by John Tindall. — 2nd ed., corr. and augm. — London: Sold by Robert Fenn ..., 1834. — viii, 231p, [1] leaf of plates: ill; 18cm (12mo)
Subscribers' names: p.225-231

630 Tindall's Yorkshire farriery: being a treatise on the diseases of horses ... / by John Tindall. — Huddersfield: Printed and sold by J. Lancashire ... sold also by Longman, Hurst, Rees, Orme and Brown ... London ..., 1814. — [8], vii, [8]-227, [14]p; 22cm (8vo)
Subscribers' names: p.[229-240]
Errata: p.[8]

TOPHAM, Thomas
631 A new compendious system on several diseases incident to cattle: wherein the disorders are orderly described ... / by Thomas Topham. — York: Printed by L. Pennington ... and sold by Scatcherd and Whitaker ... and T. Scollick ... London, 1787. — xvi, 432p; 23cm (8vo)
List of subscribers: p.422-432
Two leaves of ms notes inserted
Smith considers the name Thomas Topham to have been a pseudonym; the earliest edition of this work which he describes is a London imprint of 1788

TOWNSHEND, James

632 The royal farrier; or, the art of farriery display'd: in which is pointed out and particularly described the numerous diseases and accidents to which that most useful animal a horse, is subject ... / by James Townshend ... — London: Printed for Isaac Fell ..., [17--]. — vi, [2] (blank), 158p; 18cm (12mo)
Noted in Rothamsted (which suggests the date 1771) but not otherwise recorded. Not in BL or NUC; not known to Smith or to Huth; not in RVC or RCVS

633 **A TREATISE ON THE USEFULNESS OF FURZE OR GORSE, AS WINTER FEED FOR CATTLE**: but principally for horses ... / Translated from the Welch. — London: Longman and Co. ..., 1834. — 18p; 18cm (12mo)
Translated from the Welsh
Apparently unrecorded: not in BL, NUC, Rothamsted, Southampton, Smith, Fussell, RVC or RCVS

TREMBLEY, Abraham, 1710-1784

634 The art of hatching and bringing up domestic fowls, by means of artificial heat: being an abstract of Monsieur de Reaumur's curious work upon that subject; communicated to the Royal Society, in January last / by Mr. Trembley ...; Translated from the French. — London: Printed for C. Davis ..., 1750. — [2], 61p; 20cm (8vo)

TROWELL, Thomas

635 The Kentish farrier: wherein are contain'd the best approved medicines ... / by Thomas Trowell, of Tenterden in Kent. — London: Printed for R. Wilkin ..., 1728. — [4], 97, [10]p: ill; 20cm (8vo)
Errata: p.[4]

TRYON, Thomas, 1634-1703

636 The country-man's companion: or, a new method of ordering horses & sheep: so as to preserve them both from diseases and casualties ... / by Philotheos Physiologus ... — London: Printed and sold by Andrew Sowle ..., [1684]. — [8], 173, [3]p; 14cm (8vo)
By Thomas Tryon
Reference: Wing T3176

TURNER, James, d.1860

637 A treatise on the foot of the horse: and a new system of shoeing, by one-sided-nailing ... / by James Turner. — London: Printed for the author; and published by Longman, Rees, Orme, Brown, Green, and Longman, 1832. — xii, 106p; 26cm (8vo)
A collection of papers from the Veterinarian

TUSSER, Thomas, 1524?-1580

638 Five hundred points of good husbandry: as well for the champion or open countrey, as also for the woodland or several, mixed in every moneth, with houswifery, over and besides the book of houswifery / newly set forth by Thomas Tusser, gent. — Corrected, better ordered and newly augmented ... — London: Printed by T.R. and M.D. for the Company of Stationers, 1672. — 146, [3]p; 19cm (4to)
Reference: Wing T3369
Copy 1: Imperfect: last [3]p missing. Cropped
Copy 2: Imperfect: p.[1]-8 missing. Bound with: An essay in order to fix the nature and cure of the distemper now raging among the horned cattle / by a physician. — Lincoln: J. Rose, [1747?] Ms. notes

TWAMLEY, J. (Josiah)

639 Essays on the management of the dairy: including the modern practice of the best districts in the manufacture of cheese and butter ... / by J. Twamley, and others. — A new edition, corrected and enlarged. — London: Printed for J. Harding ..., 1816. — xi, [1] (blank), 178p: ill; 18cm (12mo)
G.E. Fussell's copy (signature)
Reference: Fussell, II, 132

USHER, John

640 Border breeds of sheep / by John Usher. — Kelso: J. & J.H. Rutherford, 1875. — vi, [2], 76, 28p; 16cm
Advertisements on 28p at end

VALE, W. (William)

641 A manual of poultry diseases / by W. Vale. — London: Published by Alex. Comyns, [1888]. — viii, [9]-98p; 19cm

642 Profitable poultry: how to manage fowls, turkeys, ducks & geese in health and disease / by W. Vale; illustrated by F.J.S. Chatterton. — 2nd ed. — London: Printed by J.D. Smith, [1896?]). — [4], 130p: ill, port; 23cm
Imprint from colophon

VEGETIUS RENATUS, Publius

643 [Ars veterinaria] Vegetii Renati Artis veterinariae, sive Mulomedicinae libri quatuor ... — Basileae: Excudebat Ioannes Faber Emmeus Iuliacensis, 1528. — [8], 72 leaves; 19cm (4to)
Imprint from colophon

644 [Ars veterinaria] Pub. Vegetii viri illustris Mulomedicina: ex trib. vetustiss. codd. varietate adiecta ... / opera Ioan. Sambuci Pannonij. — Basileae: Per Petrum Pernam, 1574. — [15], 4-196p; 23cm (4to)
References: Adams V342; Wellcome (pre-1641) 6525
Bound with: Ton 'Ippiatrikon biblia duo = Veterinariae medicinae libri duo. — Basileae: Apud Ioan. Valderum, 1537

645 [Ars veterinaria] Vegetii Renati Artis veterinariae sive Mvlomedicinae libri qvatvor / cvrante Jo. Matthia Gesnero. — Mannhemii: Cura & sumptibus Societatis Literatae, 1781. — 370p; 17cm (8vo)

646 [Ars veterinaria. English] Vegetius Renatus Of the distempers of horses: and of the art of curing them ... / translated into English by the author of the translation of Columella. — London: Printed for A. Millar ..., 1748. — xxxi, [1], vi, [7]-421, [3]p; 20cm (8vo)
Illustration: page 154

VETERINARY COLLEGE, LONDON

647 A brief examination of the views of the Veterinary College: and of the grounds of their petition presented to the House of Commons. — London: Printed for Debrett ... and Egerton ..., 1795. — [4], 36p; 21cm (8vo)
This anonymous pamphlet was not known to either Smith or Pugh. The author stresses the importance of the Petition submitted to, and currently being considered by, the House of Commons in 1795 for financial help to secure completion and permanency for the Veterinary College, London. This was of national importance not only to reduce the cost of preventable diseases in animals, but also to provide trained veterinarians for the British cavalry. The Petition was successful and the College received £1,500 annually from 1795 to 1813 (Pugh p.95-99). Provenance: J.W. Barber-Lomax
Illustration: page 155

648 Veterinary College, London: established April 8, 1791, for the reformation and improvement of farriery, and the treatment of cattle in general. — London: Printed by James Phillips ..., 1791. — 15, [1]p; 16cm (8vo)
This early version of the Proposed regulations of the Veterinary College, London was not known to Smith nor apparently to Pugh (p.36-65). The pocket booklet of 15 pages covers the constitution, management, and teaching programme for the proposed College which was formally announced in March of the same year. The first course of lectures began in January 1792

VIAL DE SAINT BEL, Charles
see SAINBEL, Charles Vial de, 1753-1793

W., J.
see WORLIDGE, John

WALKER, John
649 The botfly of the ox (oestrus bovis); or Warbles in hides: their history, life, ... / by John Walker. — London: T.C. Jack, 1886. — 15, [20]p; ill; 19cm
Advertisements on [20]p at end

WALLIS, Thomas, surgeon
650 The farrier's and horseman's complete dictionary: containing the art of farriery in all its branches ... / by Thomas Wallis ... — London: Printed for W. Owen ... and E. Baker, at Tunbridge Wells, 1759. — vi, [330]p; 18cm (8vo)

VEGETIUS RENATUS

OF THE

DISTEMPERS of HORSES,

And of the

ART of CURING them:

AS ALSO

Of the DISEASES of OXEN, and of the REMEDIES proper for them;

AND

Of the beft Method to preferve them in Health, and reftore them when fick, and to prevent the Spreading and Communication of Infectious Diftempers, according to the Practice of the ancient *Romans*.

Tranflated into *Englifh* by the Author of the Tranflation of *Columella*.

PROVERBS xii. ℣. 10.
A righteous Man regardeth the Life of his Beaft.

LONDON:
Printed for A. MILLAR oppofite to *Catherine-ftreet* in the *Strand*. MDCCXLVIII.

A BRIEF EXAMINATION

OF THE

VIEWS

OF THE

VETERINARY COLLEGE,

AND OF THE

GROUNDS OF THEIR PETITION

PRESENTED TO THE

HOUSE OF COMMONS.

DIGNA CERTE RES EST UT HÆC SCIENTIA EMANCI-
PETUR, ET IN SCIENTIAM SEORSUM REDIGATUR.
            BACON.

LONDON:

PRINTED FOR DEBRETT, PICCADILLY; AND EGERTON,
WHITEHALL, 1795.

651 The farrier's and horseman's complete dictionary: containing the art of farriery in all its branches ... / by Thomas Wallis ... — The third edition. — Dublin: Printed for James Williams ..., 1766. — vi, [330]p; 21cm (4to)
A2 bound behind A3

652 The farrier's and horseman's complete dictionary: containing the art of farriery in all its branches ... / by Thomas Wallis ... — The third edition. — London: Printed for J. Beecroft, [and 5 others], 1775. — vi, [330]p; 19cm (8vo)

WALLIS, Thomas, of Derby

653 The way to usefulness: or how to turn industry to advantage, containing a great number of valuable receipts ... / by Thomas Wallis. — 2nd ed. — Derby: Printed for the compiler, by G. Wilkins & Son, 1845. — 24p; 18cm (12mo)

WALTHEW, Richard

654 Artificial incubation: being the practical account of the art and science of Mr. Walthew for hatching of all kinds of poultry and game birds by steam ... / by the projector and inventor. — London: Printed for the author, 1824. — 52p; 23cm (8vo)

WATSON, Richard

655 By His Majesty's royal letters patent. R. Watson, farrier, in Norwich. His instructions for the management of horses & dogs: wherein are minutely described their several maladies ... — Third edition. — Norwich: Printed by Stevenson and Matchett, 1802. — xii, 146p; 21cm (8vo)

WATSON, Thomas

656 By His Majesty's royal letters patent, T. Watson, farrier in Norwich, His instructions for the management of horses and dogs: wherein are minutely described their several maladies ... — London: Printed by T. Harrison and S. Brooke ..., 1785. — xi, [1] (blank), 146p; 19cm (8vo)
Errata: p.[iv]
Imperfect: date of imprint cut off t.p. and first leaf missing
Smith (II, 147) refers only to the 1785 edition of this work, by J. Watson. This would appear to be a misprint for T. Watson; a testimonial letter is printed at the end of the book (p.143-146) from Wm Carr to Thomas Watson dated January 1785. The text is not changed in the 1802 edition by R. Watson except that the same testimonial letter appears addressed to Richard Watson

WEBB, James

657 The farmer's guide: or a treatise on the management of breeding-mares and cows ... / by James Webb ... — 2nd ed. — Elgin: Printed and published by A.C. Brander, 1834. — 251p; 19cm (12mo)

658 The farmer's guide: a treatise on the diseases of horses and black cattle ... / by James Webb ... — [4th ed]. — London: Blackie & Son, [18--]. — 223p, [3] leaves of plates: ill; 19cm (8vo)

The two titles by Webb are the same work with only the title changed in the later edition. Both copies are ex G.E. Fussell

WEBSTER, Richard W.
659 The practical management of poultry with a view to profit: a guide to successful poultry keeping on a large or small scale / by Richard W. Webster. — London: Simpkin, Marshall, Hamilton, Kent & Co., 1899. — [12], 146p, [11] leaves of plates: ill; 19cm

WEIR, Harrison, 1824-1906
660 Our poultry and all about them: their varieties, habits, mating, breeding, selection and management for pleasure and profit ... / by Harrison Weir. — London: Hutchinson, [1903]. — 2v (viii, 442p, [53] leaves of plates; vii, [1], 443-822p, [31] leaves of plates): ill (some col.); 28cm

WESTON, R. (Richard), 1733-1806
661 Tracts on practical agriculture and gardening: particularly addressed to the gentlemen-farmers in Great Britain ... To which is added, a chronological catalogue of English authors on agriculture, botany, gardening, &c. / by R. Weston, esq. ... — The second edition, greatly improved. — London: Printed for S. Hooper ..., 1773. — iv, XXXI, [1] (blank), 298, [2], 136p, [1] leaf of plates: ill ; 21cm (8vo)
Reference: Fussell, II, 85

WHITE, James, d. 1825?
662 The anatomy and physiology of the horse's foot: concisely described; with practical observations on shoeing ... / by James White ... — London: Printed for T. Chapman ..., 1801. — xvi, 160, [1]p, 13 [i.e.14] leaves of plates: ill (some col.); 15cm (12mo)
Of this first publication of James White (1801), Smith (III, 95) states, "No copy of this work is in existence, so far as we are aware"
Illustration: page 158

663 A compendious dictionary of the veterinary art: containing a concise explanation ... / by James White ... — London: Printed for Longman, Hurst, Rees, Orme, and Brown [and 4 others], 1817. — [4], 344p, [1] folded leaf of plates: ill; 18cm (12mo)

664 A compendium of cattle medicine: or, practical observations on the disorders of cattle ... / by James White. — 6th ed / re-arranged, with copious notes and additions, by W.C. Spooner. — London: Longman, Brown, Green, and Longmans ... [and 6 others], 1842. — xvi, 322p, [1] leaf of plates: ill; 22cm (8vo)

665 A compendium of the veterinary art: containing an accurate description of all the diseases to which the horse is liable ... / by James White ... — Canterbury: Printed by W. Bristow, for J. Badcock ..., London, 1802. — vi, [7]-20, 232p, 14 [i.e. 15] leaves of plates: ill (some col.); 19cm (12mo)

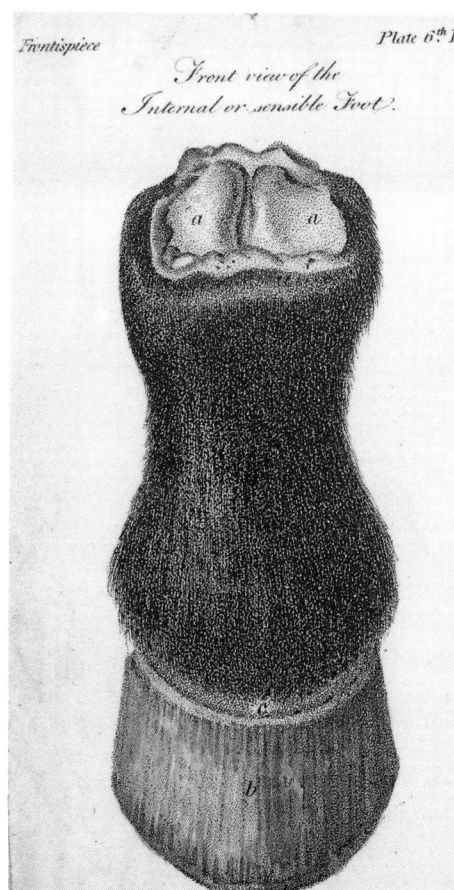

Frontispiece. Plate 6th Fig 1st.
Front view of the Internal or sensible Foot.

THE ANATOMY AND PHYSIOLOGY
OF
THE HORSE'S FOOT,
CONCISELY DESCRIBED;

WITH

Practical Observations on Shoeing;

TOGETHER WITH

The Symptoms of, and most approved Remedies for,

THE DISEASES OF HORSES.

WITH FOURTEEN ILLUSTRATIVE PLATES.

Dedicated by Permission to
THE PRESIDENT, COMMITTEE, AND MEMBERS
Of the Commercial Travellers' Society.

BY JAMES WHITE,
Veterinary Surgeon to his Majesty's First, or Royal Dragoons.

LONDON:
PRINTED FOR T. CHAPMAN, 151, FLEET-STREET.
By T. Gillet, Salisbury-square.

1801.

666 A compendium of the veterinary art: containing an accurate description of all the diseases to which the horse is liable ... / by James White ... — London: Printed for J. Badcock ... and W. Bristow, Canterbury, [1802?]. — xii, 234, xiii, [1]p, 14 [i.e.15] leaves of plates: ill (some col.); 19cm (12mo)

667 A compendium of the veterinary art: containing an accurate description of all the diseases to which the horse is liable ... / by James White ... — The sixth edition, corrected. — London: Printed for J. Badcock ... and W. Bristow, Canterbury; and sold by Longman and Co. ..., [1804?]. — 2v (vii, [1], 234, xvii, [1]p, 14 leaves of plates; ix, [3], 262, [2]p): ill (some col.); 19cm (12mo)
Vol.2: The materia medica and pharmacopoeia. — London: Printed for John Badcock ... by J.D. Dewick ..., 1804

668 A treatise on veterinary medicine ... / by James White, of Exeter ... — The ninth edition, considerably enlarged. — London: Printed for J. Johnson ... and Longman, Hurst, Rees and Orme ..., 1809-1811. — 2v ([8], 409, [11]p, 14 leaves of plates; [2], vii, [1], 266p): ill (some col.); 18cm (12mo)
Vol.1: Containing A compendium of the veterinary art ...; v.2: Containing The materia medica, and pharmacopoeia. A new edition, 1811
Provenance: Earl of Kintore (armorial bookplate and signatures)

669 A compendium of the veterinary art: containing plain and concise rules for the treatment of all the disorders and accidents to which the horse is liable ... / by James White ... — 13th ed. — London: Printed for Longman, Hurst, Rees, Orme, and Brown ... [and 5 others], 1820-1822. — 4v.in 2 (xlvi, 348p, [1] leaf of plates; xix, [1], 316p; xii, 288p; xv, [1], 236p, [26] leaves of plates): ill (some col.); 20cm (12mo)
Vol.1: 1822; v.2: A treatise on veterinary medicine, ... containing The materia medica, and pharmacopoeia. A new edition, 1820; v.3: A treatise on veterinary medicine ... containing Observations on the diseases of the digestive organs of the horse ... 1821; v.4: A compendium of cattle medicine ... 1821
In this copy, with the exception of the frontispiece to v.1, all the plates are bound together at the end of v.4. These include the XXIII plates listed in the Description of the plates in v.1

670 A compendium of the veterinary art: containing plain and concise rules for the treatment of all the disorders and accidents to which the horse is liable ... / by James White ... — 15th ed. — London: Printed for Longman, Rees, Orme, Brown, and Green ... [and 8 others], 1829-1831. — 3v (xlvi, 340p, 23 leaves of plates (1 folded); xii, 360p; xii, 384p, 2 leaves of plates): ill (some col.); 18cm (12mo)
Vol.2: A treatise on veterinary medicine, ... containing The materia dietetica, the materia medica, and the pharmacopoeia. 6th ed., 1831; v.3: A treatise on veterinary medicine, ... containing Practical observations on the ... digestive organs of the horse. 8th ed., 1830

WILKINSON, William
671 The modern veterinarian: with several receipts for horned cattle / by William Wilkinson. — 2nd ed. considerably enl. — Newcastle-upon-Tyne: John Clarke, 1834. — 220p; 20cm (12mo)

672 A treatise on two of the most important diseases which attack the horse: in two parts ... / by William Wilkinson ... — Newcastle: Printed by Edward Walker; Sold in London: by Longman and Co. ... by Constable and Co. in Edinburgh ..., 1818. — xiv, [2], 212p, [1] leaf of plates: ill; 27cm (4to)
List of subscribers: p.xii-xiv

WILLIAM COOPER LIMITED
673 The gardeners' and poultry keepers' guide and illustrated catalogue of goods manufactured and supplied / by W. Cooper Ltd. — London: William Cooper Ltd., [1913?]. — 638p: ill; 19cm
Cover title

WILLIAMSON, E. F.
674 Every farmer his own farrier and cattle doctor / [by E.F. Williamson]. — [S.l.: s.n., 1890?]. — 31, [1]p; 18cm
An advertising booklet for Fields' cattle oils, blood balls, blood powders, and pig powders, manufactured by E.F. Williamson, manufacturing and export chemist

WILSON, Yorick
675 The gentleman's modern system of farriery, or stable directory: a concise treatise on the various diseases of horses ... / by Yorick Wilson ... — Trenton: Printed and published by James Oram, 1811. — iv, [5]-95p; 19cm (12mo)
This American edition reprinted from The gentleman's veterinary monitor, and stable guide ... by Yorick Wilson, ... of Leamington. — London, 1809

WINGFIELD, W.
676 The poultry book: comprising the characteristics, management, breeding, and medical treatment of poultry ... / by W. Wingfield, G.W. Johnson; with coloured representations ... by Harrison Weir. — London: Orr, 1853. — iv, [3], 324p, [22] leaves of plates: col. ill; 26cm
The plate listed as at p.226 is incorporated onto that at p.155. The plate listed as at p.288 is incorporated onto that at p.295. There is an additional plate of Black Polands with White Crests at p.158 which is not listed

WINTER, James W., d. 1886
677 The horse: in health and disease ... / by James W. Winter. — London: Parry & Co., 1852. — viii, 376p, [1] leaf of plates: ill; 23cm

WOOD, David
678 Sheep-dipping: a digest of the latest information ... / by David Wood. — 3rd ed. — Edinburgh: Macniven & Cameron, 1893. — xi, [1], 66p: plan; 18cm

WOOD, John
679 A new compendious treatise of farriery: wherein are set forth in a plain, familiar, and natural manner the disorders incident to horses ... / by John Wood ... — London: Printed for the author, at Mr. Hewett's ... and sold by J. Brindley ... [and 3 others], 1757. — xiv, [15]-28, [2], xcviii, 136, 6, 72p; 21cm (8vo)

The names of the subscribers: p.[15]-28
Bound with: A supplement to the New compendious treatise / by John Wood. — London: Mr. Hewett's, 1758

680 A supplement to the New compendious treatise of farriery: concerning inflammations, tumours ... / by John Wood ... — London: Printed for the author, at Mr. Hewett's ... [and 3 others], 1758. — [?], 88p; 21cm (8vo)
Bound with: A new compendious treatise / by John Wood. — London: Mr. Hewett's, 1757

681 A new compendious treatise of farriery: wherein are set forth in a plain, familiar, and natural manner, the disorders incident to horses ... / by John Wood ... — The second edition. — London: Printed for J. Ryall ..., 1762. — xii, lvii, 141, [1] (blank), 62p, [2] leaves of plates: ill; 18cm (12mo)
Two plates have been added for this second edition: a frontispiece of the skeleton of a horse and, facing the first page of text, a plate of a hoof and shoe

WOOD, T. B. (Thomas Barlow), 1869-1929
682 Bullock feeding experiments in Norfolk / by T.B. Wood. — [S.l.: s.n., 1899]. — 24p; 22cm
Reprinted from the Journal of the Board of Agriculture, vol.6, 1899, p.311-332

WORLIDGE, John
683 Systema agriculturae; the mystery of husbandry discovered: treating of the several new and most advantagious ways of tilling, planting, sowing ... to which is added Kalendarium rusticum ... and Dictionarium rusticum ... / published for the common good: by **J.W.** gent. — The second edition carefully corrected and amended ... — London: Printed by J.C. for Thomas Dring ..., 1675. — [35], 324, [4]p: ill; 30cm (fol.)
Added engraved t.p. Kalendarium rusticum and Dictionarium rusticum have special title pages
By John Worlidge
Provenance: G.E. Fussell (signature)

WORSHIPFUL COMPANY OF POULTERS
684 The Charter of the Worshipful Company of Poulters, London: its orders, ordinances, and constitution: also Acts granted by the Corporation of London, with a list of the estates and charities belonging to and under the direction of the Court of Assistants of the said Company. — [London: The Company, 1871]. — vii, [1], 81p; 25cm

WRIGHT, G. H. C.
685 The farmers' veterinary guide ... / compiled by G.H.C. Wright; edited by F. Tonar. — 5th ed. / rev. and enl. by a Fellow of the Royal College of Veterinary Surgeons. — Edinburgh: Turnbull & Spears, [1894]. — xi, 113p; 19cm
The treatise to which was awarded the prize of £30 offered by the Proprietor of the "Farming World" for the best treatise on the ailments of farm live stock

WRIGHT, Lewis, 1838-1905

686 The Brahma fowl: a monograph / by Lewis Wright. — 3rd and rev. ed. — London: Cassell, Petter and Galpin: Journal of Horticulture and Cottage Gardener, 1873. — 144p, [4] leaves of plates: ill. (some col.); 19cm

687 The illustrated book of poultry: with practical schedules for judging, constructed from actual analysis of the best modern decisions / by Lewis Wright. — Rev. ed. — London: Cassell, [1886?]. — viii, 591p, [50] leaves of plates: ill (some col.); 29cm

688 The new book of poultry / by Lewis Wright. — London: Cassell, 1902. — vii, 600p, [46] leaves of plates: ill (some col.); 28cm

689 The practical pigeon keeper / by Lewis Wright. — Twelfth thousand. — London: Cassell, [1895]. — vi, [2], 232p: ill; 19cm
Originally published: 1879

690 The practical poultry keeper: a complete and standard guide to the management of poultry, whether for domestic use, the markets, or exhibition / by L. Wright. — 5th ed. — London: Cassell, Petter, and Galpin, [1872?]. — viii, 252p, [12] leaves of plates: ill (some col.); 19cm

691 The practical poultry keeper: a complete and standard guide to the management of poultry whether for domestic use, the markets, or exhibition / by L. Wright. — 20th ed. — London: Cassell, 1885 (1895 printing). — viii, 247p, [8] leaves of plates: ill (some col.); 19cm

692 The practical poultry keeper / by Lewis Wright. — New ed. — London: Cassell, 1905 (1917 printing). — viii, 315p, [8] leaves of plates: ill.(some col.); 19cm
First ed. published: 1867

WYKE, Isaac

693 The English and Welsh cattle doctor ... / by Isaac Wyke ... = Y meddyg anifeiliaid Saesonaeg a Chymraeg ... / gan Isaac Wyke ... — [Abergavenny]: Printed for and sold by I. Wyke, and Wm. Stucley, Abergavenny, [1812]. — [6], 173p; 23cm (8vo)
Date from English catalogue of books
Parallel English and Welsh text
Not known to Smith or to Fussell; not in RVC or RCVS. See Ashton, G.M. (1973) Early books in Welsh on veterinary medicine. Veterinary history, 2, 13-23 (who suggests a date of c.1820)
Illustration: page 163

YOUATT, William, 1776-1847

694 Cattle: their breeds, management, and diseases / [by W. Youatt]. — London: Baldwin and Cradock, 1842. — viii, 600p: ill; 23cm (8vo). — (Library of useful knowledge)
Published under the superintendence of the Society for the Diffusion of Useful Knowledge

THE ENGLISH AND WELSH CATTLE DOCTOR:

CONTAINING
A CONCISE, YET AN ACCURATE DESCRIPTION, OF THE
DIFFERENT DISORDERS
TO WHICH
HORNED CATTLE, CALVES, SHEEP, AND SWINE,
ARE MOST LIABLE;
WITH
THE BEST METHODS OF TREATMENT
HITHERTO KNOWN.

By *ISAAC WYKE*,
APOTHECARY, CHEMIST, AND DRUGGIST.
The Welsh Part by an able Translator.

Y MEDDYG ANIFEILIAID
SAESONAEG A CHYMRAEG:
YN CYNNWYS DARLUNIAD CRYNO A CHYWIR O'R
AMRYWIOL ANHWYLIADAU
I BA RAI Y MAE
DA CORNIOG, LLOI, DEFAID A MOCH,
YN FWYAF AGORED,
YNGHYD
A'R MODDION GOREU O DRINIAETH
AG SYDD HYD YN HYN YN ADNABYDDUS.

Gan *ISAAC WYKE*,
FLERYLLYD, A GWERTHWR, MODDION MEDDYGOL.
Y Rhan Gymraeg gan Gyfieithydd.

Printed for and Sold by
I. WYKE, and WM. STUCLEY, Abergavenny.
Price 5s. in Boards.

695 The complete grazier: or, farmer's and cattle breeder's and dealer's assistant ... / by William Youatt. — 9th ed., enl. ... / by M.A. Youatt. — London: Cradock and Co., 1852. — [4], viii, 718p: ill; 23cm

696 The dog / by William Youatt. — London: Charles Knight, 1848. — [8], 268p: ill; 23cm (8vo)
At head of title: Under the superintendence of the Society for the Diffusion of Useful Knowledge

697 The horse: with a treatise on draught ... / [by W. Youatt]. — London: Baldwin and Cradock, 1837. — viii, 472p: ill; 23cm (8vo). — (Library of useful knowledge)
Published under the superintendence of the Society for the Diffusion of Useful Knowledge
On the title page of a New edition of The horse ... published by Edward Law, London, 1858, it is stated that the Treatise on draught was written by I.K. Brunel, C.E., F.R.S., the engineer

698 The pig: a treatise on the breeds, management, feeding, and medical treatment of swine ... / by William Youatt; illustrated with engravings drawn from life by William Harvey. — London: Cradock and Co., 1847. — viii, 164p: ill; 24cm (8vo)

699 The pig / by William Youatt. — 2nd ed. / enl. and re-written by Samuel Sidney. — London: Routledge, Warne, & Routledge, 1860. — xiv, [2], 260p, 16 leaves of plates: ill, plans; 20cm

700 Sheep: their breeds, management, and diseases. To which is added The mountain shepherd's manual / [by W. Youatt]. — London: Baldwin and Cradock, 1837. — viii, 568, 36p: ill; 23cm (8vo). — (Library of useful knowledge)
Published under the superintendence of the Society for the Diffusion of Useful Knowledge

701 Sheep: their breeds, management, and diseases / by William Youatt ...; to which are added, remarks on the breeds and management of sheep in the United States, and on the culture of fine wool in Silesia. — New York: C.M. Saxton, 1862. — 159, [1]p: ill; 24cm
Published under the superintendence of the Society for the Diffusion of Useful Knowledge

YOUNG, Arthur, 1741-1820
702 An essay on the management of hogs: including experiments on rearing and fattening them ... — London: Printed for W. Nicoll ..., 1769. — xxiv, 3-49p; 17cm (8vo)
By Arthur Young
Believed to be the first published work in English devoted entirely to pigs. The BL notes editions of 1769 and 1770, and these entries are quoted by Amery; but not known to Smith or to Fussell, not in RVC or RCVS
Illustration: page 165

AN ESSAY
ON THE
MANAGEMENT OF HOGS;
INCLUDING
EXPERIMENTS
ON
REARING AND FATTENING THEM:

FOR WHICH

The SOCIETY for the Incouragement of ARTS, MANUFACTURES, and COMMERCE, adjudged the PREMIUM of a

GOLD MEDAL.

LONDON:

Printed for W. NICOLL, N° 51, in St. Paul's Church Yard.

MDCCLXIX.

703 [The farmer's guide. French] Le guide du fermier: ou instructions pour élever, nourrir, acheter & vendre les bêtes à cornes ... — A Paris: Chez J.P. Costard ..., 1770. — 2v ([4], 263, [1]; [4], 262p); 17cm (12mo)
Translation of the 4th ed. of The farmer's guide by Arthur Young

704 The farmer's kalendar; or, a monthly directory for all sorts of country business: containing, plain instructions ... / by an experienced farmer. — London: Printed for Robinson and Roberts ... and J. Knox ..., 1771. — [32], 399p; 21cm (8vo)
By Arthur Young. Cf. BLC, v.358, p.36

Reference books

705 The **AGRICULTURAL MERCHANT.** — Downham Market: John Powling Farm Seeds, [19--]. — 20p: port; 25cm
Facsim. of Vol.1, no.1 (June 1920)

ALDER, Garry
706 Beyond Bokhara: the life of William Moorcroft. Asian explorer and pioneer veterinary surgeon, 1767-1825 / Garry Alder. — London: Century, 1985. — xiii, 417p, [8]p of plates: ill, maps, ports; 24cm

707 **AMERICAN POULTRY HISTORY, 1823-1973**: an anthology overview of 150 years, people-places-progress / by the American Poultry Historical Society; Oscar August Hanke editorial director ... — Madison: The Society, 1974. — 775p: ill, ports; 24cm

AMERY, G. D.
708 The writings of Arthur Young / by G.D. Amery. — London: Royal Agricultural Society of England, 1925. — 31p; 22cm
Cover title
From the Journal of the Royal Agricultural Society of England, vol.85, 1924

709 **ANIMAL HEALTH**: a centenary, 1865-1965: a century of endeavour to control diseases of animals. — London: HMSO, 1965. — xviii, 396p, [24]p of plates: ill, maps, ports.; 25cm
At head of title: Ministry of Agriculture, Fisheries and Food

ARBER, Agnes
710 Herbals: their origin and evolution: a chapter in the history of botany, 1470-1670 / by Agnes Arber. — 2nd ed. rewritten and enl. — Cambridge: At the University Press, 1938 (1953 printing). — xxiv, 325p, xxvi leaves of plates: ill, ports; 24cm

ARNOLD AND SONS
711 Catalogue of veterinary appliances, &c. / Arnold & Sons. — London: Arnold & Sons, 1902. — 88p: ill; 25cm

712 A catalogue of veterinary instruments / manufactured and sold by Arnold and Sons. — London: Arnold and Sons, 1874. — 56, [16]p: ill; 22cm

713 Catalogue of veterinary instruments / manufactured by Arnold and Sons. — London: Arnold and Sons, 1886. — xi, 153, [3]p: ill; 21cm

714 Catalogue of veterinary instruments / manufactured by Arnold & Sons. — London: Arnold & Sons, 1893. — [8], viii, 216p: ill; 25cm

715 Catalogue of veterinary instruments and appliances / Arnold & Sons. — London: Arnold & Sons, 1900. — viii, xvi, 365p: ill; 25cm

716 Catalogue of veterinary instruments and appliances / Arnold & Sons. — London: Arnold & Sons, [1901]. — [8], viii, 303p: ill; 29cm

717 Veterinary instruments, &c / Arnold & Sons, (John Bell & Croyden, Ltd.). — London: Arnold and Sons, [1905?]. — [16], 171p: ill; 29cm

BAILEY, Jocelyn
718 The village blacksmith / Jocelyn Bailey. — 2nd ed. — Aylesbury: Shire Publications, 1980 (1983 printing). — 32p: ill, coat of arms, ports; 21cm. — (Shire album; 24)
Previous ed.: 1977

BAILLIÈRE, TINDALL AND COX
719 List of veterinary works (including books for agricultural students) and periodicals / published and sold by Baillière, Tindall and Cox. — London: Baillière, Tindall and Cox, 1914, 1925. — 2v; 19cm

BARANSKI, Anton
720 Geschichte der Thierzucht und Thiermedicin im Alterthum / Anton Baranski. — Hildesheim: Georg Olms, 1971. — viii, 245p; 21cm
Facsim. reprint of: Wien: W. Braumüller, 1886

BARBER, R. H. (Robert Heberden), 1916-
721 A supplementary bibliography of hawking: being a catalogue of books published in England between 1891 and 1943 ... / by R.H. Barber. — Westminster: Priv.print.for the author by W. Hay Fielding & Co., Ltd., 1943. — [15]p; 21cm

BATH AND WEST AND SOUTHERN COUNTIES SOCIETY
722 Catalogue of the library / compiled by Peter Pagen, Philip Bryant. — Bath: [The Society], 1964. — 86p, [1] leaf of plates: ill; 22cm

BENNION, Elisabeth
723 Antique medical instruments / Elisabeth Bennion. — London (Russell Chamber, Covent Garden, W.C.2): Philip Wilson Publishers Ltd for Sotheby Parke Bernet Publications, 1979. — xiii, 355p, fold leaf, [16]p of plates: ill(some col); 26cm

BLISS AND CO.
724 Export catalogue – of – modern saddlery, harness, horse clothing, &c. — London: Bliss & Co., [1910?]. — 51 leaves: chiefly ill. (some col.); 21x28cm
Introduction dated: October, 1910
Cover title

BOLTON, Henry Carrington

725 A catalogue of scientific and technical periodicals, 1665-1895: together with chronological tables and a library check-list / by Henry Carrington Bolton. — 2nd ed. — City of Washington: Smithsonian Institution, 1897. — vii, 1247p; 24cm. — (Smithsonian miscellaneous collections; v.40)

726 **BRITISH BEEF CATTLE.** — Bletchley: Meat and Livestock Commission, Beef Improvement Services, 1976. — 48p: col.ill.; 30cm

BRITISH MUSEUM

727 Guide to an exhibition of manuscripts and printed books illustrating the history of agriculture. — [London]: Printed for the Trustees [of the British Museum], 1927. — 30p, VIII leaves of plates: ill, facsims; 25cm

BRITTEN, James

728 Old country and farming words: gleaned from agricultural books / by James Britten. — London: Published for the English Dialect Society by Trubner & Co., 1880. — xvii, 191p; 23cm

BROWNE, Charles A. (Charles Albert)

729 A source book of agricultural chemistry / by Charles A. Browne. — Waltham, Mass.: Chronica Botanica, 1944. — x, 290p: ill, facsims.; 26cm. — (Chronica botanica; v.8, no.1)

BUTTRESS, F. A. (Frederick Arthur), 1908-

730 Agricultural periodicals of the British Isles, 1681-1900, and their location / compiled by F.A. Buttress. — Cambridge: University of Cambridge, School of Agriculture, 1950. — 15p; 21cm

COLLINS, E. J. T. (Edward John T.)

731 Sickle to combine: a review of harvest techniques from 1800 to the present day / by E.J.T. Collins. — Reading: Museum of English Rural Life, University of Reading, 1969. — 47p: ill, facsims, maps; 29cm

COMBEN, N. (Norman)

732 The early English printed literature on the diseases of poultry and other birds / N. Comben. — Oxford: Pergamon Press, 1969. — 11p, [2]p of plates: facsims; 25cm
Repr. from The Veterinarian, v.6, p.17-25

733 The **CURE IN 1800** ...: a collection of some old veterinary remedies. — Wilmslow: Imperial Chemical (Pharmaceuticals) Limited, [1952]. — [12] leaves: ill; 28cm
Cover title
Letter from the publisher laid in

DANMARKS VETERINAER- OG JORDBRUGSBIBLIOTEK

734 Fortegnelse over boger om heste 1530-1773 i Danmarks veterinaer-og jordbrugsbibliotek / udarbejdet af Ivan Katic og Karen Geert Kristiansen. — [S.l.: s.n.], 1974. — 24p; 23cm
Offprint from: Nordisk veterinaermedicin, 1974, v.26, suppl.3

DENHAM, Sidney

735 Cats between covers: a bibliography of books about cats / by Sidney Denham; with a foreword by Sir Compton Mackenzie. — London: Published by H. Denham, 1952. — 44p; 22cm

DIRCKS, H. (Henry), 1806-1873

736 A biographical memoir of Samuel Hartlib: Milton's familiar friend; with bibliographical notices of works published by him; and a reprint of his pamphlet entitled "An invention of engines of motion" / by H. Dircks. — London: John Russell Smith, 1865. — x, 124p; 20cm

EDWARDS, Everett E. (Everett Eugene)

737 A bibliography of the history of agriculture in the United States / by Everett E. Edwards. — Washington: United States Government Printing Office, 1930. — 307p; 23cm. — (Miscellaneous publication / United States Department of Agriculture; no.84)
G.E. Fussell's copy (signature)

738 A bibliography on the agriculture of the American Indians / compiled by Everett E. Edwards and Wayne D. Rasmussen. — Washington: United States Government Printing Office, 1942. — 107p; 23cm. — (Miscellaneous publication / United States Department of Agriculture; no.447)
G.E. Fussell's copy (signature)

EGERTON, Judy

739 George Stubbs, anatomist and animal painter / Judy Egerton ; [photographs by A.C. Cooper Ltd et al.]. — London: Tate Gallery Publications, 1976. — 64p, plate: ill, 1port; 25cm
With essay by Basil Taylor and some of the catalogue notes by David Brown. — Accompanies an exhibition held at the Tate Gallery 25 August-3 October 1976
Includes extracts from Ozias Humphry's 'Memoir of George Stubbs'

[The FANCIER'S GAZETTE]

740 Ross Poultry Ltd. and Poultry world present the 100th anniversary issue of the Fancier's gazette. — [S.l.]: Poultry world, 1974. — 20p: ill; 30cm
Facsim. of Vol.1, no.1 (Apr.11, 1874), issued as suppl. to Poultry world

FREEMAN, B. M. (Barry Metcalfe)

741 A short history of the Houghton Poultry Research Station / B.M. Freeman and J.F. Tucker. — Houghton: The Station, 1984. — v, 68p; 21cm

FUSONIE, Alan M.
742 Heritage of American agriculture: a bibliography of pre-1860 imprints / compiled by Alan M. Fusonie. — Beltsville, Md.: National Agricultural Library, 1975. — iv, 71p; 26cm. — (Library list; no.98)
G.E. Fussell's copy (inscription)

FUSSELL, G. E. (George Edwin)
743 Agricultural history in Great Britain and Western Europe before 1914: a discursive bibliography / G.E. Fussell. — London: Pindar, 1983. — 157p; 22cm

744 The English dairy farmer: 1500-1900 / G.E. Fussell. — London: Frank Cass & Co., 1966. — 357p, [12]p of plates: ill; 22cm

745 The farmers tools, 1500-1900: the history of British farm implements, tools and machinery before the tractor came / by G.E. Fussell. — London: Andrew Melrose, 1952. — 246p, 111p of plates: ill; 23cm

746 Farming history and its framework / G. E. Fussell. — [Davis, Calif.: Agricultural History Society], [197-]. — p.132-146; 22cm
A reprint from Agricultural history

747 More old English farming books: from Tull to the Board of Agriculture, 1731 to 1793 / G.E. Fussell. — London: Crosby Lockwood & Son, 1950. — vii, 186p, viiip of plates: ill, facsims, port.; 22cm
Signed by the author
Generally referred to as Vol. 2

748 The old English farming books: from Fitzherbert to Tull 1523 to 1730 / G.E. Fussell. — London: Crosby Lockwood & Son, 1947. — 141p, 16p of plates: ill, facsims, port; 22cm
Signed by the author
Generally referred to as Vol. 1

749 Old English farming books, 1523-1793: Fitzherbert to the Board of Agriculture / G.E. Fussell. — Collieston: Aberdeen Rare Books, 1978. — 141, v, 186p, [1] leaf of plates: port; 22cm
Facsim. reprints of: The old English farming books. — London: C. Lockwood, 1947; and: More old English farming books. — London: C. Lockwood, 1950
No.4 of a limited edition of 500. Signed by the author

750 The old English farming books / G.E. Fussell. Vol.3: 1793-1839. — London: Pindar, 1983. — 285p; 22cm
Signed by the author

751 The old English farming books / G.E. Fussell. Vol 4: 1840-1860. — London: Pindar, 1984. — 115p; 23cm

752 Short-title catalogue of the library of works illustrative of the history of agriculture in all its branches: held by G.E. Fussell ... as at end-1983. — [S.l.: s.n., 1984]. — 45 leaves; 30cm
Cover title

753 **G.E. FUSSELL**: a bibliography of his writings on agricultural history. — Reading: Museum of English Rural Life, University of Reading, 1967. — vii, 34p; 24cm

GILBEY, Sir Walter, 1831-1914
754 Catalogue of the fine library of sporting literature formed by Sir Walter Gilbey, Bart ...: sold by auction by Messrs. Christie, Manson & Woods ... June 21, 1915 ... — London: Christie, Manson & Woods, 1915. — 82p; 25cm

GITTINS, Nigel
755 Charles Vial de Sainbel, sa vie – son oeuvre / par Nigel Gittins. — [Paris: N. Gittins, 1984]. — 79p; 21cm
Thesis (doctorat vétérinaire) — École nationale vétérinaire d'Alfort, 1984

GRAY, Ernest A.
756 The trumpet of glory: the military career of John Shipp, first veterinary surgeon to join the British Army / by Ernest A. Gray. — London: Hale, 1985. — 127p, [4]p of plates: ill, 1plan, 2facsims; 23cm

GREAT BRITAIN. Commissioners of Patents
757 Patents for inventions. Abridgments of specifications relating to agriculture: Division I. Field implements (including methods of tilling and irrigating land) A.D. 1618-1866. — London: Commissioners of Patents for Inventions, 1876. — xvii, 929p; 20cm

758 Patents for inventions. Abridgments of specifications relating to agriculture: Division I. Field implements (including methods of tilling and irrigating land), part II – A.D. 1867-1876. — London: Commissioners of Patents, 1878. — xvi, 492p; 19cm

GREAT BRITAIN. Patent Office. Library
759 Subject list of works on agriculture, rural economy, and allied sciences: in the Library of the Patent Office. — London: Patent Office, 1905. — 424p; 16cm. — (Patent Office Library series; no.15). — (Bibliographical series; no.12)
Imperfect: t.p. missing. Ms letter laid in

GRIMSHAW, Anne
760 The horse: a bibliography of British books 1851-1976: with a narrative commentary on the role of the horse in British social history, as revealed by the contemporary literature / Anne Grimshaw. — London: Library Association, 1982. — xxxiv, 474p: ill, 1port; 26cm
No.144 of limited edition of 1000 signed copies

HALL, Sherwin A.
761 The cattle plague of 1865 / by Sherwin A. Hall. — [London: Dawsons of Pall Mall], 1962. — p.45-58; 25cm
Reprinted from Medical history, v.6, no.1, 1962

HAMS, Fred
762 Old poultry breeds / Fred Hams. — Aylesbury: Shire Publications, 1978. — 32p: ill; 21cm. — (Shire album; 35)
Ill. on inside front cover

HARTING, James Edmund, 1841-1928
763 Bibliotheca accipitraria: a catalogue of books ancient & modern relating to falconry ... / by James Edmund Harting. — London: Holland Press, 1964. — xxviii, 289p, [26] leaves of plates: ill, ports.; 23cm
Originally published: London: Quaritch, 1891

HARVEY, John, 1911-
764 Early gardening catalogues: with complete reprints of lists and accounts of the 16th-19th centuries / by John Harvey. — Chichester: Phillimore, 1972. — xii, 182, [14]p of plates (1 folded): ill, facsims; 23cm

HAUSSMANN AND DUNN
765 Headquarters for veterinary books / Haussmann & Dunn. — Chicago: Haussmann & Dunn, [1900]. — 15p: ill; 23cm

HENDERSON, I. F. (Isabella Ferguson)
766 A dictionary of scientific terms: pronunciation, derivation, and definition of terms in biology, botany, zoology, anatomy, cytology, embryology, physiology / by I.F. Henderson and W.D. Henderson. — Edinburgh: Oliver and Boyd, 1920. — viii, 354p; 23cm

HENREY, Blanche
767 British botanical and horticultural literature before 1800 : comprising a history and bibliography of botanical and horticultural books printed in England, Scotland, and Ireland from the earliest times until 1800 / Blanche Henrey. — London: Oxford University Press, 1975. — 3v (xxvi, 290p, [1] leaf of plates; xvi, 748p, 30, [1] leaves of plates (1 folded); xvii, 142p, [1] leaf of plates): ill(some col), facsims, plans, ports(1 col); 28cm

HENRY WOOLDRIDGE AND SONS
768 [Catalogue of] self-fastening frost cogs and steel-headed frost nails ... / Henry Wooldridge & Sons. — Lye, Stourbridge: Henry Wooldridge & Sons, 1939. — 24p: chiefly ill.; 29cm

769 A **HISTORY OF THE OVERSEAS VETERINARY SERVICES.** — London: British Veterinary Association, 1961-1973. — 2v; 24cm
Pt.1 edited by G.P. West

HUBBARD, Clifford
770 An introduction to the literature of British dogs: five centuries of illustrated dog books / by Clifford L.B. Hubbard. — Ponterwyd: Published by the author, 1949. — viii, 56p, 11 leaves of plates: ill, facsim., ports.; 22cm

HUTH, F. H. (Frederick Henry)
771 Works on horses and equitation: a bibliographical record of hippology / by F.H. Huth. — London: B. Quaritch, 1887. — x, 439p; 22cm

INGRAM, Arthur
772 The country animal doctor / Arthur Ingram. — Aylesbury: Shire Publications, 1979. — 32p: ill; 21cm. — (Shire album; 40)

INTERNATIONAL BEE RESEARCH ASSOCIATION
773 British bee books: a bibliography, 1500-1976 / by International Bee Research Association; principal collaborators Joan P. Harding ... [et al.]. — London (Hill House, Gerrards Cross, Bucks, SL9 0NR): The Association, 1979. — 270p: ill, facsims; 22cm

J. BIBBY AND SONS LTD.
774 The Bibby story: this booklet has been specially produced to commemorate the centenary of J. Bibby & Sons Ltd. — 2nd impression. — Liverpool: J. Bibby & Sons Ltd., 1978. — 32p: col.ill.; 25cm
Designed, written and produced by Robinson Lees Design Associates

J.H.H. AND CO. LTD.
775 Illustrations. — [S.l.]: J.H.H. & Co. Ltd., [19--?]. — 39 leaves: chiefly ill. (some col.); 28cm
"Sole manufacturers: – Hawkins Limited" – p.32A

JOSEPH BRECK AND SONS
776 Illustrated catalogue of poultry supplies / Joseph Breck & Sons. — 17th ed. — Boston: J. Breck & Sons, 1913. — 24p: ill; 28cm

KESTER, Wayne O.
777 The history of the American Association of Equine Practitioners 1954-1979 / by Wayne O. Kester. — Golden, Colo.: The Association, 1980. — vi, 160p: ill, ports.; 23cm

KIRKNESS, J. M.
778 A history of the Animal Health Register / J.M. Kirkness. — London: The Association of the British Pharmaceutical Industry, 1982. — 39p: ports; 21cm

KONGELIGE VETERINAER- OG LANDBOHOJSKOLE. Bibliotek
779 Katalog over den Kongelige Veterinaer- og landbohojskoles bibliotek: indtil udgangen af 1894. — Kobenhavn: I kommission hos Aug.Bang., 1898. — xlvi, 888p; 24cm

KROHNE AND SESEMANN

780 Catalogue of veterinary instruments / manufactured and sold by Krohne & Sesemann ... — London: [Krohne & Sesemann], 1889. — 116p: ill; 26cm

LECLAINCHE, Emmanuel

781 Histoire illustrée de la médecine vétérinaire / Emmanuel Leclainche; presentée par Gaston Ramon. — [S.l.]: Editions Albin Michel, 1955. — 2v: ill; 32cm

LIBRAIRIE AGRICOLE DE LA MAISON RUSTIQUE

782 Librairie agricole de la maison rustique, rue Jacob, 26, à Paris : [catalogue]. — Paris: Librairie agricole, 1888. — 48p; 19cm

LINDLEY LIBRARY

783 The Lindley Library: catalogue of books, pamphlets, manuscripts and drawings. — London: Royal Horticultural Society, 1927. — vii, 487p; 25cm

MACDONALD, Gilbert

784 In pursuit of excellence: one hundred years Wellcome: 1880-1980 / [written by Gilbert Macdonald]. — London: Wellcome Foundation, 1980. — 120p: ill(some col.), ports; 25cm
Author's presentation copy

MADDEN, E.

785 Brucellosis: a history of the disease and its eradication from cattle in Great Britain / [E. Madden]. — [London]: Ministry of Agriculture, Fisheries and Food, 1983. — 81, [1]p: 6maps; 24cm
Foreword by W.H.G. Rees, dated Jan.1984 is inserted
Cover title

MATOLCSI, János

786 Hungarian Agricultural Museum / János Matolcsi. — Debrecen: Mezögazdasági Könyvkiadó, 1967. — 15p, [34]p of plates: ill; 23cm

MCDONALD, Donald

787 Agricultural writers: from Sir Walter of Henley to Arthur Young, 1200-1800 ... / by Donald McDonald. — London: Horace Cox, 1908. — 228p; 27cm

MENNESSIER DE LA LANCE, Gabriel René

788 Essai de bibliographie hippique: donnant la description détaillée des ouvrages publiés ou traduits en latin et en français sur le cheval et la cavalerie ... / par le général Mennessier de la Lance. — Paris: L. Dorbon, 1915-1921. — 2v. + suppl.; 25cm

MORGAN, Raine
789 Farm tools, implements and machines in Britain: pre-history to 1945: a bibliography / by Raine Morgan. — [Reading]: Institute of Agricultural History, University of Reading: British Agricultural History Society, c1984. — xxii, 275p; 21cm. — (Bibliographies in agricultural history; no.3)

MORTON, Sholto Charles John Hay Douglas, Earl of
790 The Chelsea Physic Garden. — A 2nd ed. rev. and augm. / by The Earl of Morton ... — London: [Trustees of the London Parochial Charities], 1973. — [16]p: col.ill; 24cm + 1 booklet (7p, maps; 21cm)

MUSEUM OF ENGLISH RURAL LIFE
791 Portraits of animals: a catalogue of the nineteenth century paintings and prints of farm livestock in the Museum of English Rural Life. — Reading: The Museum, 1964. — 39p; 33cm

792 The **MUSEUM OF VETERINARY HISTORY AT SKARA**: tillkommet på initiativ av Sveriges Veterinärförbund. — [Skara]: Rådet för veterinärhistorisk och biografisk forskning, [1981]. — 6p; 21cm
Cover title

NORRIS, John E.
793 Books on poultry and cock-fighting: a collectors bibliography / by John E. Norris. — Paoli, Pa.: J.E. Norris, 1977. — 33p; 23cm

OXFORD, Arnold Whitaker
794 English cookery books to the year 1850 / by Arnold Whitaker Oxford. — London: Henry Frowde, Oxford University Press, 1913. — 192p; 19cm

PALMBY, Clarence D., 1916-
795 Made in Washington: food policy and the political expedient / Clarence D. Palmby. — Danville, Ill.: Interstate Printers & Publishers, c1985. — xi, 226p: ill., ports.; 24 cm
Author's presentation copy

PATTISON, Iain, 1914-1991
796 The British veterinary profession 1791-1948 / Iain Pattison. — London: J.A. Allen, 1984. — x, 207p, [4]p of plates: 1facsim, ports; 23cm
Two copies; one, 1983 printing, withdrawn as defective; annotated by the author

797 John McFadyean: a great British veterinarian / by Iain Pattison. — London: J.A. Allen, 1981. — 240p: 1port; 23cm
Author's presentation copy

PEARL, M. L. (Morris Leonard)
798 William Cobbett; a bibliographical account of his life and times / by M. L. Pearl; with a foreword by G. D. H. Cole. — Westport, Conn.: Greenwood Press, [1971]. — vii, 266 p; 23 cm
Reprint of the 1953 ed

PERKINS, Walter Frank
799 British and Irish writers on agriculture / compiled by W. Frank Perkins. — 2nd ed. — Lymington: Printed and published by Chas. T. King, 1932. — ix, 193p; 22cm

PODESCHI, John B.
800 Books on the horse and horsemanship: riding, hunting, breeding & racing 1400-1941 / a catalogue compiled by John B. Podeschi. — London: Tate Gallery for the Yale Center for British Art, 1981. — xvii, 427p, [18] leaves of plates: ill(some col.), 2maps, music, facsims, 1plan, ports (some col.), 1geneal.table; 30cm. — (The Paul Mellon collection) (Sport in art and books)

POLLARD, Alfred William, 1859-1944
801 A short-title catalogue of books printed in England, Scotland, & Ireland: and of English books printed abroad, 1475-1640 / compiled by A.W. Pollard & G.R. Redgrave; with the help of G.F. Barwick ... [et al.]. — London: Bibliographical Society, 1926 (1956 printing). — xviii, 609p; 26cm

PORTER, Joshua
802 Catalogue of books on agriculture and rural affairs: being part of the stock of Joshua Porter, agricultural bookseller ... — Dublin: [J. Porter, 1828?]. — 8p; 20cm

803 **[POULTRY LITERATURE].** — [London: J. Murray, 1851]. — p.[317]-351; 23cm
Extracted from: Quarterly review, vol.88, p.[317]-351

POYNTER, F. N. L.
804 A bibliography of Gervase Markham, 1568?-1637 / by F.N.L. Poynter. — Oxford: Oxford Bibliographical Society, 1962. — vi, 218p, 4 leaves of plates: facsims; 26cm. — (Oxford Bibliographical Society publications; new series, vol.11)
Revision of thesis (PhD.) — University of London
Author's presentation copy

805 **PRINTING AND THE MIND OF MAN**: assembled at the British Museum and at Earls Court, London, 16-27 July 1963. — [London]: F.W. Bridges & Sons: Association of British Manufacturers of Printers' Machinery, c1963. — 125, 61p, 32, 16p of plates: ill, facsims; 24cm
Organised in connexion with the 11th International Printing Machinery and Allied Trades Exhibition
Pt.2 has separate t.p. with subtitle: An exhibition of fine printing in the King's Library of the British Museum, July-September 1963

PUGH, L. P.
806 From farriery to veterinary medicine, 1785-1795 / by L.P. Pugh. — Cambridge: Published for the Royal College of Veterinary Surgeons by W. Heffer and Son, 1962. — xiii, 178p, XXIVp of plates: ill, facsims., ports.; 24cm

PUNNETT, R. C. (Reginald Crundall)
807 Notes on old poultry books / by R.C. Punnett; with a bibliography up to 1880 by E. Comyns Lewer and R.C. Punnett. — London: "The Feathered World", 1930. — 40p, [1] leaf of plates: facsim; 22cm

REID LIBRARY
808 Catalogue of books on agriculture, in the Reid Library, Rowett Research Institute: which were formerly in the libraries of Sir Archibald Grant of Monymusk, Collingwood Lindsay Wood of Freeland, and others / compiled by J.C.R. Yeats. — Bucksburn, Aberdeen: The Library, 1961. — 19, iii leaves; 27cm

ROHDE, Eleanour Sinclair
809 The old English gardening books / by Eleanour Sinclair Rohde. — London: Martin Hopkinson and Co., 1924. — xii, 144p, XVI leaves of plates: ill, port, facsims; 25cm. — (The new Aldine library; 5)

810 The old English herbals / by Eleanour Sinclair Rohde. — London: Longmans, Green and Co., 1922. — xii, 243p, [18] leaves of plates: ill; 26cm

ROTHAMSTED EXPERIMENTAL STATION. Library
811 Catalogue of the printed books on agriculture: published between 1471 and 1840. With notes on the authors / by Mary S. Aslin. — [Harpenden: The Station, 1926]. — 331p, [19] leaves of plates: facsims.; 26cm

812 Library catalogue of printed books and pamphlets on agriculture: published between 1471 and 1840 / Librarian: Mary S. Aslin. — 2nd ed. — Harpenden: The Station, 1940. — 293p, [1] leaf of plates; 25cm

813 Prints and paintings of British farm livestock, 1780-1910: a record of the Rothamsted collection / by D.H. Boalch; with an historical sketch ... by John Hammond. — Harpenden: Rothamsted Experimental Station Library, 1958. — xxxiv, 126p, XXXII p of plates: ill; 25cm

814 Supplement to the library catalogue of printed books and pamphlets on agriculture: published between 1471 and 1840. List of additions since 1940. — [Harpenden: The Station], 1949. — 15p; 24cm

ROYAL AGRICULTURAL SOCIETY OF ENGLAND. Library
815 Catalogue of the library of the Royal Agricultural Society of England. — London: The Society, 1918. — iv, 386p; 24cm
"The catalogue is the work of G.E. Manwaring" — Introd.

ROYAL COLLEGE OF VETERINARY SURGEONS. Library

816 Catalogue of modern works, 1900-1954: with a section showing periodicals and reports. — London: Royal College of Veterinary Surgeons, 1955. — 98p; 22cm + 2 suppl. (16p, 14p)
At head of title: Royal College of Veterinary Surgeons Memorial Library
Supplements are for 1955-6 and 1957-8

817 Catalogue of the historical collection: books published before 1850. — London: Royal College of Veterinary Surgeons, 1953. — 36p; 22cm
At head of title: Royal College of Veterinary Surgeons Library

ROYAL VETERINARY COLLEGE. Library

818 A catalogue of the books, pamphlets and periodicals up to 1850 / with an introduction by L.P. Pugh. — [London]: Royal Veterinary College Library, 1965. — 48p; 21cm
Supplement to the Veterinary record, May 1st 1965

819 The **ROYAL VETERINARY COLLEGE AND HOSPITAL**: this brochure has been prepared to commemorate the opening of the Royal Veterinary College by His Majesty King George VI at 11.30 a.m. on Tuesday November 9th, 1937 ... — London: [The College], 1937. — 46p: ill, port.; 29cm
G.E. Fussell's copy (signature)

S. MAW AND SON

820 Book of illustrations to S. Maw & Son's quarterly price-current. — London: S. Maw & Son, 1869. — [4], 241p: ill; 27cm

S. MAW, SON AND THOMPSON

821 Book of illustrations to S. Maw, Son & Thompson's quarterly price-current: surgeons' instruments, etc. — London: S. Maw, Son & Thompson, 1891. — x, 235p: ill; 27cm

SCHLEBECKER, John T.

822 Bibliography of books and pamphlets on the history of agriculture in the United States 1607-1976 / John T. Schlebecker. — Santa Barbara, Calif.: ABC-Clio, 1969. — vii, 183p; 25cm
Author's presentation copy to G.E. Fussell

SMITH, Sir Frederick, 1857-1929

823 The early history of veterinary literature and its British development / by Sir Frederick Smith. Vol.1: From the earliest period to A.D.1700. — London: Baillière, Tindall and Cox, 1919. — iv, 373p, [8] leaves of plates: ill, facsims, ports; 25cm
Repr. from the Journal of comparative pathology and therapeutics, 1912-1918
Photocopy

824 The early history of veterinary literature and its British development / by Sir Frederick Smith. Vol.1: From the earliest period to A.D.1700. — London: J.A. Allen & Co., 1976. — iv, 373p, [8] leaves of plates: ill, facsims, ports; 25cm
Repr. from the Journal of comparative pathology and therapeutics, 1912-1918. — Facsim. reprint of: London: Baillière, Tindall and Cox, 1919

825 The early history of veterinary literature and its British development / by Sir Frederick Smith. Vol.2: The eighteenth century. — London: Baillière, Tindall and Cox, 1924. — viii, 244p; 25cm
Repr. from the Veterinary journal, 1923-24

826 The early history of veterinary literature and its British development / by Sir Frederick Smith. Vol.2: The eighteenth century. — London: J.A. Allen & Co., 1976. — viii, 244p; 25cm
Repr. from the Veterinary journal, 1923-24. — Facsim. reprint of: London: Baillière, Tindall and Cox, 1924

827 The early history of veterinary literature and its British development / by Sir Frederick Smith. Vol.3: The nineteenth century, 1800-1823. — London: Baillière, Tindall and Cox, 1930. — vii, 184p, VI leaves of plates: ill, ports; 25cm
Repr. from the Veterinary journal, 1929-1930

828 The early history of veterinary literature and its British development / by Sir Frederick Smith. Vol.3: The nineteenth century, 1800-1823. — London: J.A. Allen & Co., 1976. — vii, 184p, VI leaves of plates: ill, ports; 25cm
Repr. from the Veterinary journal, 1929-1930. — Facsim. reprint of: London: Baillière, Tindall and Cox, 1930

829 The early history of veterinary literature and its British development / by the late Sir Frederick Smith. Vol.4: The nineteenth century, 1823-1860 / edited, with a memoir of the author, by Fred Bullock. — London: Baillière, Tindall and Cox, 1933. — xxiv, 161p, XII leaves of plates: ports; 25cm
Editor's presentation copy

830 The early history of veterinary literature and its British development / by the late Sir Frederick Smith. Vol.4: The nineteenth century, 1823-1860 / edited, with a memoir of the author, by Fred Bullock. — London: J.A. Allen & Co., 1976. — xxiv, 161p, XII leaves of plates: ports; 25cm.
Facsim. reprint of: London: Baillière, Tindall and Cox, 1933

831 A history of the Royal Army Veterinary Corps: 1796-1919 / by Sir Frederick Smith. — London: Baillière, Tindall and Cox, 1927. — x, 263p, [1], XIII leaves of plates: ill (some col.), ports.; 25cm

SMITH, R. N. (Richard Norman)
832 Dr. J.A. MacBride, M.R.C.V.S., itinerant professor extraordinary / R.N. Smith. — [London]: Veterinary History Society, 1980. — [12]p: facsims; 30cm
Cover title

SMITHCORS, J. F.
833 Evolution of the veterinary art: a narrative account to 1850 / by J.F. Smithcors. — Kansas City: Veterinary Medicine Publishing Co., 1957. — xvii, 408p: ill; 24cm
Author's presentation copy to Norman Comben. Letter from the author to N. Comben laid in

SPARKES, Ivan G. (Ivan George)
834 Old horseshoes / Ivan G. Sparkes. — Aylesbury: Shire Publications, 1976. — 32p: ill; 21cm. — (Shire album; 19)
Ill. on inside front cover

SPARROW, Walter Shaw
835 British farm animals in prints and in paintings / by Walter Shaw Sparrow. — London: Walker's Galleries, 1932. — 50p, [22] leaves of plates: ill; 22cm. — (Walker's quarterly; nos.33-34)

STAUGAARD, H. C.
836 Mund- og klovesyge / af H.C. Staugaard. — 2. opl. — København: Veterinaermedicinsk museum den Kgl. Veterinaer- og Landbohøjskole, 1982. — 15p: ill; 24cm

STUBBS, George, 1724-1806
837 George Stubbs 1724-1806. — London: Tate Gallery Publications, 1984. — 248p: ill(some col.), ports; 34cm: cased
Catalogue of an exhibition at the Tate Gallery 17 October 1984-6 January 1985 and at the Yale Centre for British Art, 13 February-7 April 1985

TOOLE STOTT, Raymond
838 Circus and allied arts: a world bibliography 1500-1957: based mainly on circus literature in the British Museum, the Library of Congress, the Bibliotheque Nationale and on his own collection / by R. Toole Stott; with a foreword by M. Willson Disher. — Derby: Harpur & Sons (Derby) Ltd distributors, 1958-1971. — 4v: ill; 27cm
Dates in subtitles vary

TROW-SMITH, Robert
839 A history of British livestock husbandry to 1700 / Robert Trow-Smith. — London: Routledge and Kegan Paul, 1957. — x, 286p, [16]p of plates: ill; 22cm

840 A history of British livestock husbandry 1700-1900 / Robert Trow-Smith. — London: Routledge and Kegan Paul, 1959. — x, 351p, 24p of plates: ill; 22cm

UNITED STATES. National Agricultural Library
841 Historic books and manuscripts concerning general agriculture in the collection of the National Agricultural Library / [compiled by Mortimer L. Naftalin]. — Washington, D.C.: The Library, 1967. — 94p; 26cm. — (Library list; no.86)
G.E. Fussell's copy (signature). T.p. missing and photocopy supplied

UNIVERSITY OF READING. Institute of Agricultural History
842 Guide to the Institute of Agricultural History and Museum of English Rural Life. — Reading: University of Reading, 1982. — 122p in various pagings; 30cm
Two copies; one Part 6, Paintings and prints, only

UNIVERSITY OF READING. Library
843 Accessions of historical farm records revised up to March 1970. — [Reading]: University of Reading, 1970. — 20 leaves; 30cm
Caption title
G.E. Fussell's copy (signature)

844 Accessions of historical farm records up to December 1967. — [Reading]: University of Reading, 1968. — 12 leaves; 30cm
Caption title

845 Historical farm records: a summary guide to manuscripts and other material in the University Library collected by the Institute of Agricultural History and the Museum of English Rural Life. — Reading: University of Reading, Library, 1973. — xii, 320p; 25cm

UNIVERSITY OF SOUTHAMPTON. Library
846 Catalogue of the Walter Frank Perkins agricultural library. — Southampton: The University Library, 1961. — xii, 291p, [1] leaf of plates: port; 25cm

847 **VETERINARY HERITAGE** / bulletin of the American Veterinary History Society. — [S.l.: The Society], 1983-1986. — 28cm
Holdings: Vol.6, no.2 (Apr.1983) — v.9, no.2 (Aug.1986)

WALKER, Robin E.
848 Ars veterinaria: l'art vétérinaire de l'antiquité à la fin du XIXeme siècle: essai historique / Robin E. Walker. — Levallois- Perret: Galena, 1972. — 85p: ill (some col.), facsims; 27cm
No.125 of a limited ed. of 250

WHITE, K. D. (Kenneth Douglas), b.1908
849 A bibliography of Roman agriculture / by K.D. White. — Reading: University of Reading, 1970. — xxviii, 63p; 24cm. — (Bibliographies in agricultural history; no.1)

WILLIAM ALLDAY AND CO.
850 Sectional catalogue of "Alcosa": British made blowers, portable forges ... — Birmingham: William Allday & Co. Ltd., [1922?]. — 58p: ill; 22cm

WILSON, Andrew
851 A history of the Yorkshire Veterinary Society 1863-1980 / by Andrew Wilson. — [S.l.: s.n., 1981?]. — 52p; 21cm
Cover title

WILSON, Sir Graham
852 The Brown Animal Sanatory Institution / by Graham Wilson. — Cambridge: Cambridge University Press, 1979. — p.155-176, 337-352, 501-521, 171-197; 23cm
Reprinted from the Journal of hygiene, v.82-83, 1979

853 **WORLD DIRECTORY OF AGRICULTURAL LIBRARIES & DOCUMENTATION CENTRES** / edited by D.H. Boalch. — Harpenden, Herts: International Association of Agricultural Librarians & Documentalists, 1960. — 280p; 24cm

WORSHIPFUL COMPANY OF FARRIERS
854 The farriers of London: being an account of the Worshipful Company of Farriers as described in the records of the company / compiled by Leonard C.F. Robson. — [London]: Printed by order of the Court for private circulation, 1949. — 203p, [6] folded leaves of plates: ill, facsims.; 23cm

WRIGHT, Lucille N.
855 Books on poultry husbandry / compiled by Lucille N. Wright. — Ithaca, N.Y.: James E. Rice Memorial Poultry Library, 1961. — 79p; 23cm. — (Publication / James E. Rice Memorial Poultry Library; no.2)

WYE COLLEGE. Library
856 A catalogue of agricultural & horticultural books, 1543-1918, in Wye College Library. — Ashford, Kent: The Library, [1977]. — [1], ii, 100p; 30cm

YOUNG, Arthur, 1741-1820
857 Catalogue of valuable books and manuscripts: including the library of the late Arthur Young, esq. F.R.S. ... which will be sold by auction, by Messrs. Sotheby, Wilkinson & Hodge ... 1st of December, 1896 ... — London: Sotheby, Wilkinson & Hodge, 1896. — 100p; 25cm

YOUNG AND CO.
858 Cow house fittings, piggery fittings, and stable fittings, &c., &c. / Young & Co. — London: Young & Co., [191-]. — 64p: ill; 27cm
Cover title

859 Young's stable and cowhouse fittings ... — [London]: Young and Co., [between 1929 and 1932]. — 176p: ill; 29cm
Price list dated 1932 laid in

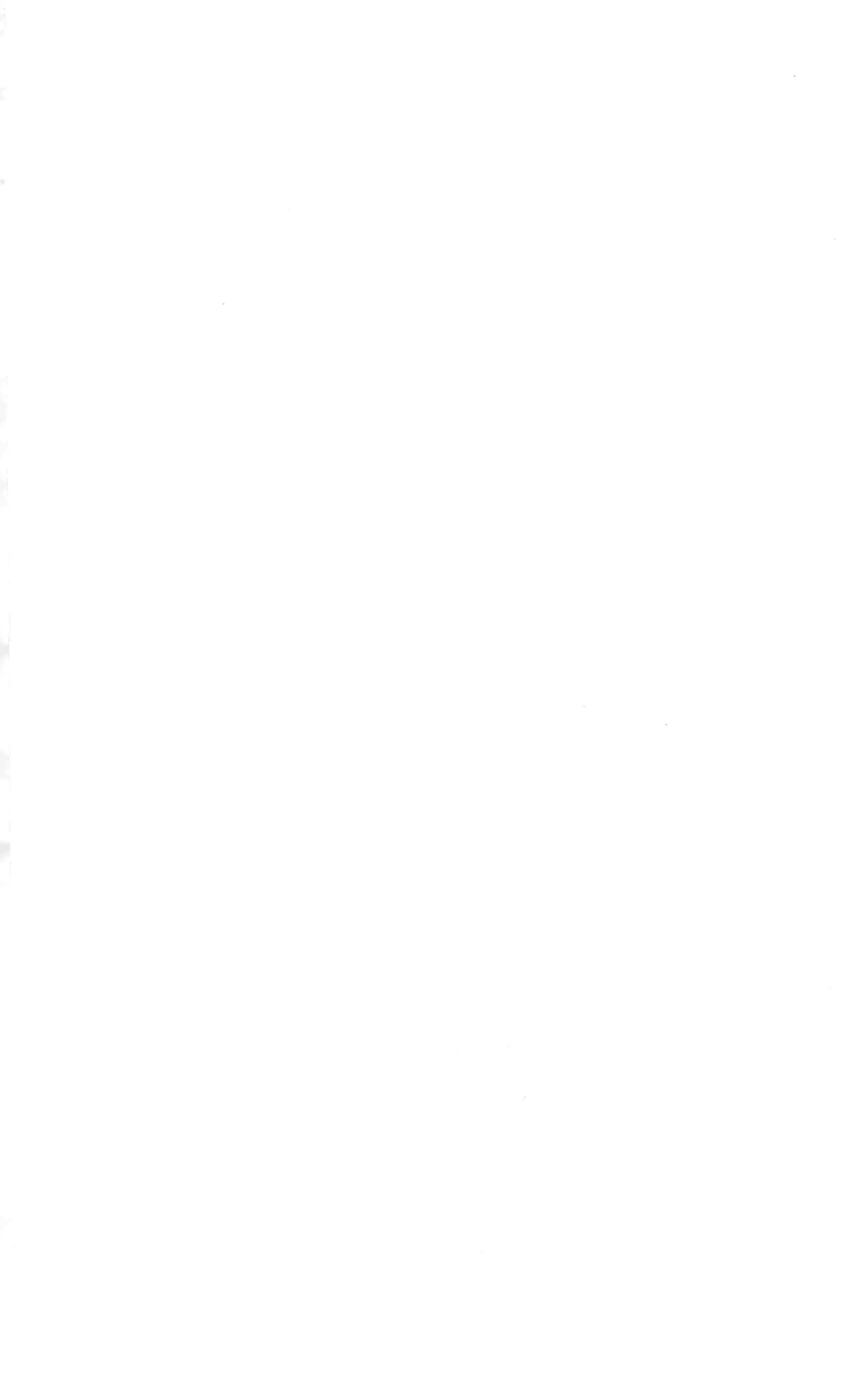